THE ART
OF
HEALTH

Your Health Warrior Awakens

THE ART

OF

HEALTH

Your Health Warrior Awakens

A 12-Week Program to Achieve Optimal Health,
Based on the Principles of Sun Tzu

Dr. Kevin Chan
with
Penny Breen Aleo

Copyright

To my beloved wife Josephine (from whom I still have a lot to learn), my family, and my children - Elliott, Isabelle, and Ethan, especially Elliott.

TABLE OF CONTENTS

Foreword

Introduction

Week 12

Conclusion

THE ART OF HEALTH

Your Health Warrior Awakens

FOREWORD

Healthcare is perhaps one of the most controversial topics of the modern era. It has caused numerous bankruptcies and even premature deaths. It would seem only warfare has caused more suffering. Although many in the healthcare industry -- hospitals, insurance, and drug companies -- are trying to solve its problems, few are able to offer viable solutions. When entities' profits are dependent upon sick people needing expensive medications and services, it is easy to see the conflict of interest in their efforts.

Unless you have a family member in the healthcare industry, it is difficult to find someone who is fully interested in your health and well-being. Fortunately, Dr. Kevin Chan, whose book is in your hands, is such a doctor. He sincerely cares about educating people about their health, and offers wise, innovative, and effective approaches to significantly improve their life.

Dr. Chan was our honored speaker at the 2016 Inaugural Sun Tzu's *Art of War* Conference at Vanderbilt University. His knowledgeable speech, which educated us on how to stay healthy, left us speechless because the information he shared was so different from what we thought to be true. Armed with his philosophy and proposal of healthcare, as it pertains to the timeless Sun Tzu's *Art of War*, we all felt that the healthcare industry as a whole is more than ready for a positive change.

As the founder of Sonshi, the preeminent resource on Sun Tzu's *Art of War* since 1999, I have met many accomplished scholars and practitioners of the Chinese classic over the years, including professionals from all areas, generals, billionaires, and celebrities. Yet Dr. Kevin Chan stands out. He and I have spoken at length regarding the subject of health. His ideas are smart and creative, yet grounded in real-world experience. More importantly, in every discussion, his focus has always been on excellent patient care and sincerely helping people lead a healthier life.

If Sun Tzu was a doctor, I believe he would think like Dr. Chan, and many ailments and diseases would be soundly defeated. Dr. Chan's advice on health focuses on practical actions that are strategic, holistic, and root-cause seeking. He advocates approaches that are preventative, based on simple lifestyle changes (see Weeks 3 and 4). He understands that the mind is just as important as the body, allowing our emotions to heal us instead of harming us (see Week 7). He teaches us that our environment affects us in profound ways (see Weeks 8 and 11). He even discusses the economics of healthcare and why it makes sense to do things different from the norm (see Week 2).

In summary, Dr. Chan's philosophy is balanced between advanced modern medicine and traditional approaches that work together. I am deeply grateful that *The Art of Health* is now available for all to benefit. There are few areas in life more important than health. When you get sick, it negatively affects many things in your life, including those who care about you. Thus, we must show leadership and "be a leader of your health" as Dr. Chan advises. I believe if you follow his philosophy and advise for the next 12 weeks, it may be one of the best things you ever do for yourself. The health investment you make in yourself may mean the difference between leading an unhealthy life or a healthy one.

Thomas Huynh, founder
Sonshi.com
Atlanta, GA
January 27, 2018

INTRODUCTION

"You have to believe in yourself."

~ Sun Tzu

I was around eight or nine years old when I first came across Sun Tzu's *The Art of War*. It was at that time I started to think that I wanted to become a doctor. Over the years I realized not only that I wanted to be a doctor, but that I wanted to be an innovative doctor. I wanted to do something different. Through medical school and residencies, my vision became that I not only wanted to help heal patients, but I also wanted to teach patients a philosophy about health that would add value to their lives. It is the impetus for my practice, as well as writing this book. I want to teach people how to think strategically about their health.

Many health books promote different therapies that are helpful to the authors. But, these therapies may not be helpful to others. I am not promoting specific nutritional supplements or wellness therapies, but rather a strategic system that allows you to see how pieces of health information may fit together into a bigger picture. This, in turn, helps you make better decisions about your health and your life. You decide what is right for you. In essence, this is not a book about just what to do, but how to *think* about what you should do.

We are in information overload in our society. Experts around the world agree that as we multi-task more and take in information more rapidly, there is a cognitive cost to pay. Neuroscientists at Stanford, found that information coming in while multitasking, causes the new information to go to the wrong part of the brain. Neuroscientists at MIT say our brains are not wired to quickly go from one task, and information source, to another. It increases the release of cortisol, a stress hormone, which can lead to brain damage if it remains chronically elevated.

People don't need more information; they have plenty of information at their fingertips. I feel people need strategies on how to process the information, and protocols to help them navigate life and health. I've kept Sun Tzu's principles with me throughout my life and feel they have served me, and countless others through the centuries, very well. I believe others could benefit from Sun Tzu's time-honored principles, to help them think strategically about their life and health.

There are many areas of health and medicine that I'm interested in, such as Integrative Medicine, Functional Medicine, Mind-Body Medicine, and the comparable Classical Chinese Medicine. I touch on these areas and hope to write about them in the future. But I believe the best place to begin, is to introduce an innovative way to think about medicine and health. I have always been drawn to leaders who think outside the box. I was inspired by people like Steve Jobs, someone who thought differently. I believe you must first have the right course for your thinking, before you can succeed. And I believe Sun Tzu's philosophy is one of the best courses to follow.

Sun Tzu was a gifted Chinese General and philosopher whom scholars believe wrote *The Art of War* around 2,500 years ago. It has been, perhaps, the most influential book on strategy in the world - from its inception to present day. It has been studied by world leaders in all walks of life. In the United States its competitive strategy has influenced leaders in the military, politics, business, sports and more.

"As Sun Tzu said 2,500 years ago, 'Rely not on the likelihood of the enemy's not coming, but on your own readiness to receive him; not on the chance of his not attacking, but rather on the fact that we have made our position unassailable.' This holds true for our national defense today."

~ *Robert Gates, 22nd U.S. Secretary of Defense*

"While much of our business strategy has been defined by the principles of *The Art of War*, my personal interactions have as well. In fact, Salesforce.com may never have been created, or at least would look very different, had I not followed its wisdom."

~ *Marc Benioff, Founder & CEO, Salesforce*

"As Sun Tzu said, 'Every battle is won before it's fought.' We don't have many signs around here, but that's one of the ones we have up in our locker room and meeting rooms. That's one of the few we have. I definitely believe in it."

~ *Bill Belichick, Head Coach, New England Patriots*

The Art of War is a masterpiece study of conflict on every level. It aims for victory without battle ("To win without fighting is best."). Through the psychology of conflict, insights into human nature, and complex interacting forces, the book is, and has been, a lesson in success.

As a Medical Doctor of Chinese heritage, I have studied the philosophies taught in *The Art of War* and feel they are not only relevant today, but are important in many areas of life, including health. When dealing with disease, it is better not to battle, but to prevent a battle in the first place. I have dedicated my career to teaching my patients, as well as healthcare providers and health administrators, the advantages of prevention. I feel Sun Tzu's metaphorical teachings have a lot to offer in the field of preventive medicine.

Conventional medicine is good at saving lives - that is about 20% of medicine today. The other 80% is made up of chronic illness: diabetes, cardiovascular disease, arthritis, obesity, cancer, and more. Most chronic conditions can be changed through lifestyle modifications. Conventional medicine is "sick medicine," waiting until you are sick before treatment begins. Preventive medicine is focused on prevention and requires personal responsibility from patients to adhere to a healthy lifestyle.

I have studied Sun Tzu for many years and his philosophy has been a guiding force for me, in all aspects of my life. I'm very grateful for the principles I've learned and want to share them as well as give him the honor he deserves.

His advice centers around common sense, personal responsibility, and good decision making, which I feel are lacking in our contemporary education and society today. It is my hope to help you make sense of health information so you can make better decisions. That is where   Sun Tzu comes in. Through my preventive-health guidance and Sun Tzu's common sense strategies, we can help you make better decisions for your health.

This book is not meant to be a translation, but following the chapters and advice of Sun Tzu, I will interpret his philosophies as they pertain to health. In particular, I will translate what is applicable to self-care and health coaching. I believe Sun Tzu's principles can act as a bridge for Chinese and Western medicine, especially Classical Chinese and Integrative Medicine. As you will see, according to his principles, understanding conflict (or disease) can lead not only to its resolution, but can prevent it altogether.

Sun Tzu covers 13 principles in his book. I will cover these principles in 12 chapters, as they relate to health.

SUN TZU'S 13 principles:
1. Calculations
2. Doing Battle
3. Planning Attacks
4. Formation
5. Force
6. Weakness and Strength

7. Armed Struggle
8. Nine Changes
9. Army Maneuvers
10. Ground Formation
11. Nine Grounds
12. Fire Attacks
13. Using Spies

DR. CHAN'S 13 Principles:
1. The Five Elements and Health Strategic Analysis
2. Health Economics
3. Planning the Attack: Unity and Focus
4. Health Positioning
5. Innovative Healthcare
6. Weakness and Strength in Health
7. Healthcare Direct Confrontation
8. Adaptability in Health
9. Competitive Environments in Healthcare
10. Evaluating Opportunities in Health
11. Stages of Health Situations
12. Healthcare Environmental Attacks
13. Health Information Sources

I have created 12 modules that interpret and teach Sun Tzu's 13 chapters, and also include wellness action steps. Each module is meant to be completed in one week, so that in 12 weeks you will be well on your way to optimal health.

This book can also serve as a manual to be integrated with other standard health coaching programs.

I believe the best way to approach this program is to first commit to a day and time each week when you will read the next chapter and commit to the action steps. You should also have a notebook that will become your wellness journal, where you will complete assignments and record your journey for the next 12 weeks and beyond.

To master living, you must master health. What are you willing to do for your health? If you are ready to be a wellness warrior in the art of health, then let's begin...

WEEK 1

THE FIVE ELEMENTS

AND HEALTH STRATEGIC

ANALYSIS

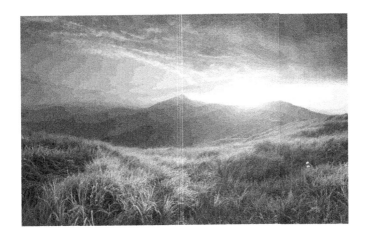

How healthy do you want to be in the future? What is your plan or strategy to get there?

Through some of Sun Tzu's most important principles, including: the Five Elements, Seven Questions, and Twelve Deceptions, this chapter teaches that we can learn through planning and strategizing. You must question the situation and honestly evaluate your weaknesses and strengths to see how you can be successful. Sun Tzu's philosophy as well as Chinese philosophy is based on comparisons: the yin and yang, being healthy and unhealthy, your health in the past, and the future. It is only through evaluating, strategizing, and planning, that you will become healthier.

Sun Tzu's lesson will be written first, and then Dr. Chan's interpretation, as it pertains to health, will follow.

1

SUN TZU said:

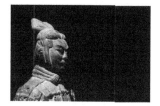

Warfare is important to a nation
It is a matter of life and death.
It is the way to survival or to destruction. So study it.

Study the five factors of warfare:
1. Way
2. Heaven
3. Ground
4. General
5. Law

Calculate your strength in each and compare them to your enemy's strengths.

The 'Way' is the strong bond your people have with you. Whether they face certain death or hope to come out alive, they never worry about danger or betrayal.

'Heaven' is dark and light, cold and hot, and the seasonal constraints.

'Ground' is high and low, far and near, obstructed and easy, wide and narrow, and dangerous and safe.

'General' is wise, trustworthy, benevolent, brave, and disciplined.

'Law' is organization, the chain of command, logistics, and the control of expenses.

DR. CHAN says:

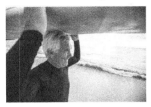

This is war against disease.
It can mean life or death.

Success depends on your relationship with Sun Tzu's Five Elements.
They are the basis of where you are and where you want to be.

The Five Elements:

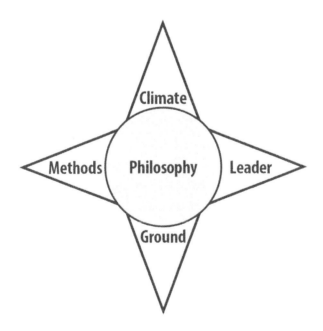

1. ***Way*** *(Mindset)*
   This is your belief system, your philosophy, your mission, and your values.

How healthy do you want to be? What do you believe? What is your mission? Your beliefs will propel you. You need to know your beliefs and values; they will lead you to a healthy life.

2. Heaven *(Mind)*

Heaven pertains to things you cannot easily control: weather, climate, the seasons, timing and trends. In health it also relates to aging. You cannot control getting older and cannot easily control changes in your body. Ask yourself – how do I deal with aging? It also pertains to your emotional wellbeing as opposed to your physical wellbeing. It pertains to Integrative medicine as opposed to conventional medicine.

3. Ground *(Body)*

This is your terrain – your body and state of physical being. It's where you have more immediate control. It's where you fight. What are you fighting for? Your health and longevity. What are you struggling with right now in your health?

4. Leader *(Character)*

The general or leader makes good decisions. Leadership pertains to things like character, personality, and attitude. Do you have what it takes to be a good leader for your health? What do you need to do or work on to be a good leader? If you are a leader of your health you must be:

- *Wise – You must be knowledgeable about your health. Study health and how you can be healthier.*
- *Trustworthy – Find good health practitioners who are trustworthy. Then do your part to be trustworthy too.*
- *Benevolent – You must have compassion and care for yourself. Health is very much about self-care.*

4

- *Courageous – You must be brave and take the actions needed to be healthy.*
- *Disciplined – Be accountable for your health. Do your part – study, have a plan, keep to your plan and follow-through.*

5. Law *(Systems)*

Systems you have set up to carry out a situation.
What systems do you have in place to keep you on your plan to becoming healthier?

What tools could you have in place to hold you accountable? You could sign up for a gym class; go through your pantry and throw out unhealthy food and only have healthy food in your home; arrange with a co-worker to walk for 15 minutes at lunch time. Put the methods in place to give yourself the support you need in becoming heathier.

Your success is determined by how well you master these elements.

SUN TZU said:

Every general has heard of these five factors - Way, Heaven, Ground, General, and Law. The one who heeds them will be victorious; the one who does not heed them will not be victorious.

Therefore, calculate and compare your levels of strength in these five factors (Way, Heaven, Ground, General, Law) to your enemy's, and determine whether you are superior.

Ask:
Which ruler has the Way?
Which general has the ability?
Which has advantage in Heaven and Ground?
Which implemented Law?
Which army is resilient?

Which officers and soldiers are trained?
Which rewards and punishes clearly?

By asking these types of questions, I know who will win and who will lose.

A general who listens to my principles and applies them, will surely be victorious; keep him.

A general who does not listen to my principles, and does not apply them, will surely be defeated; remove him.

Look for advantages when applying my principles and you will gather sufficient force to take on unforeseen situations.

Force is tilting the balance of power to your side by gathering advantages.

DR. CHAN says:

*To be successful in health you must plan and ask yourself the **Seven Inquiries**. They teach you to do the right thing at the right time. They create a method for mindfulness, e.g. eat a healthy breakfast in the morning, go to bed at a consistent time each night.*

The Seven Inquiries:

1. Do you have the right philosophy? Which healthcare provider has the right philosophy?
Find a doctor who has the healthcare philosophy that matches your healthcare philosophy.

2. Which health leader has the skill?
Which healthcare provider has the skills you need to help you become strong against disease?

*Also - **You** must be the leader of your health. Do you have the skill? You must study, practice, and create the skills needed to be healthy.*

What could you do to create the skills you need? You might research articles or ask your healthcare provider.

3. What advantages are there for mind and body?
Pick the right time and place for your health decisions. For example: Is it a good time to join a gym or will you stick to exercising if you follow a video or get on a treadmill at home after work?

4. What systems can you implement?
What methods work best for you? Do you enjoy yoga? Which will work better for you - sign up for a class or follow a yoga DVD? Walk two days a week with a friend or use your treadmill while you listen to a podcast? Pick which method works best for you to become successful.

5. Which health warrior is resilient?
What are your strengths? Play on your strengths. Are you social? Join an exercise class or a healthy cooking class. Do you like to dance? Sign up for a Zumba class at the gym or a dance class at the local dance studio. Love the outdoors? Join a hiking club and hike on the weekends.

6. Which healthcare providers have the training?
Find the providers who can help you be the healthiest you can be. Which ones have the training you are looking for? Someone trained in preventive medicine? Nutrition? Acupuncture? Find who has the best training for what you need.

7. Which rewards and consequences make sense?
The rewards of health are numerous. Good health leads to wellbeing, happiness, and longevity. Having good health gives you energy to live the life you want. Bad health leads to illness and disease. Having bad health can lead to unhappiness and a shorter life.

Which rewards and consequences make sense for you as you set up your methods for good health?

Listen to healthcare providers who have the training and can assist in helping you get healthier. Then consistently adjust your methods for greater health.

SUN TZU said:

Warfare is the Way of deception. Therefore,
> If able, appear unable
> If active, appear inactive
> If near, appear far
> If far, appear near.
> If your enemies have advantage, bait them.
> If they are confused, capture them
> If they are numerous, prepare for them
> If they are strong, avoid them
> If they are angry, disturb them
> If they are humble, make them haughty
> If they are relaxed, toil them
> If they are united, separate them.

Attack where your enemies are not prepared; go where they do not expect you to go.

This strategy leads to victory in warfare, so do not let the enemy see it.

DR. CHAN says:

The Twelve Deceptions:
Therefore, if able, appear unable
If active, appear inactive
If near, appear far
If far, appear near.

Thinking of complementary opposites can help you stay healthy. If you're healthy, it will help you stay consistently committed to a healthy lifestyle by thinking of the complementary opposite - what if you didn't live a healthy lifestyle – the unhealthy lifestyle will lead to illness.

Let me tell you my personal experience with the complementary opposite - near appears far and far appears near. My children love to go out for frozen yogurt. It is a special treat for them. If I drive to the frozen yogurt shop, it is about five minutes away, if I walk, it is about 15 minutes away. I walk the 15 minutes each way, because it is healthier to do so. But the fifteen minutes makes it feel like it is far away. It is near, but appears far.

Also, there was a church my family went to on Sundays. It is 10 minutes away, but we were always late for church. I didn't know why we were always late, always rushing to get there, until we started going to a church that is 30 minutes away. We have never been late for that church service. We know it will take 30 minutes and we allow that time and things run smoothly. But we were never on time when we went to the church 10 minutes away. It is the same principle that when something is easy or free, we don't take it seriously, we take it for granted.

This principle can also relate to intellectual closeness or distance. You may have a doctor who is right down the street, but philosophically he or she is not a good match for you. Maybe they don't use preventive strategies for their patients. They may be physically close, but intellectually distant. So you travel 30 minutes to see a doctor who is not physically close, but is philosophically a good match for you – intellectually close.

9

If your enemies have advantage, bait them – *If you have cravings for unhealthy foods, go where you know you could get it, but get something else that is healthy. Purposefully put yourself in the situation where you could have it, but don't. You will build your health muscle, so that it will not have any advantage over you.*

If they are confused, capture them – *If your family is not sure about your new healthier lifestyle, educate them, so they can join you. Studies have shown you adapt your healthy behaviors to the people around you – your peers and your family.*

If they are numerous, prepare for them - *If you have numerous signs of poor health, you must prepare yourself to get healthy. Evaluate, strategize, plan, and take action.*

If they are strong, avoid them – *If your cravings are strong for something, don't bring it in the house and don't go where you'll be tempted, until you can go and not have it.*

If they are angry, disturb them – *Your family may not like the fact that you have committed to a healthier lifestyle. They may be pretty angry that you've thrown out the junk food and are serving salads, veggies, and other healthy foods, and that you may be limiting television and computer time. They may have to be disturbed for a while until they adapt and begin to see how much better they feel.*

If they are humble, make them haughty – *If you are humble, make the commitment and let people know you are on a strong path to becoming the healthiest you can be.*

If they are relaxed, toil them - *If you are getting too relaxed with your healthy lifestyle plan, then it is time to step it up! Take it to the next level. Sign up for a class. Walk a little farther, join a hiking group, or challenge yourself to eat more veggies.*

If they are united, separate them - *If you are feeling overwhelmed with symptoms of poor health, break it down, chunk out your plan so* *you can take small steps to get healthier. Start to walk 15 minutes a day. Start to go to bed 15 minutes earlier.*

You will find a place where you can win.

The 12 deceptions play a role in your health plan – to help you fight self-sabotage and make you more adaptable and strong. Also, there is an advantage to complementary opposites, which is that you don't get too comfortable. The opposites actually enhance the qualities of each other and when you begin to live the deceptions, they make you stronger. (This is the philosophy of yin and yang, which we will learn more about in Chapter 6). Treat the situation as though you didn't lose 5 lbs., so that you don't sabotage your progress. You have to become adept in the ways of deception to prevent self-sabotage. You can be relaxed, yet still be working.

If able, remind yourself to get more training
If active, remind yourself the consequences of being inactive
If disease is near, take cautions to stay far from disease
If disease is far, remind yourself not to lower your guard as if disease is near

You can be healthy and still attract disease
You can be discouraged and still be determined
You can be qualified and still be preparing
You can be strong and still take actions to avoid getting sick
You can be frustrated and still control your emotion
You can be modest and still be confident
You can be complacent and still be disciplined
You can be close to peers and still remain independent

Yin and Yang

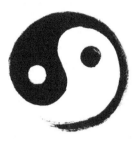

Much of Chinese philosophy is based on yin and yang. They represent the perfect balance of nature – opposite, yet interconnected forces that complement each other. There is a mutual interdependence, so that you cannot have one without the other, such as day and night and dark and light.

SUN TZU said:

Before doing battle, the one who calculates will win, because many calculations were made; before doing battle, the one who calculates but will lose, because few calculations were made.

Many calculations mean victory; few calculations mean no victory; then how much worse when there are no calculations?
From this perspective I can clearly predict victory or defeat.

DR. CHAN says:

The only way to battle disease is to claim victory over it before it even begins. That is prevention. You can calculate your advantages over disease – what makes up your preventive healthy lifestyle?

Good health care
Healthy sleep
Good nutrition
Exercise
Stress management

Strong social relationships

These advantages add up to victory. If you have only a few of these advantages, that adds up to defeat. You have to analyze your advantages to see where you are weak and strong, and then develop a plan for your success.

Wellness Warrior Actions: Week 1

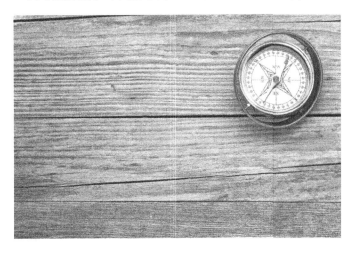

(The first week will take a bit more time than other weeks as you create your vision and go through the foundations of Sun Tzu's philosophy.)

Commit
Commit to the planning and strategies it will take to become a health warrior. Set aside a day and time each week to read the next chapter and complete the Wellness Warrior Actions.

The Five Elements, Seven Questions and Twelve Deceptions
Using your journal, write Week 1 at the top of the page and go back and read through Dr. Chan's interpretations of the Five Elements, Seven Questions, and Twelve Deceptions. Attempt to use the Five Elements Model to depict your current unique strategic health position. Answer any questions in the sections and write your observations about how they relate to your life and health. Pick one

area of your health that you could focus on as you answer the different questions and make your observations.

Vision meditation
- Have your journal ready to record your thoughts after you meditate.
- Sit in a private, quiet, and comfortable place.
- Close your eyes and relax.
- Take a deep breath in and exhale three times to empty the air in your chest (this will start your deep breathing).
- Take a breath for each number as you count backwards from 10 to 1, as you relax your body and center yourself. Notice where there is tension and let it go with your breath.
- **For Week 1** - Begin to see who you would like to be in the future, a few months from now, a year from now, 10 years from now. See yourself as very healthy. What does that look like? What does that feel like?

Journaling:
- Write "Week 1 – My Vision" in your journal, then begin to write the vision you see for your healthy future self. What do you see yourself doing? How do you feel? What else is happening in your life in your vision? Write everything you want in your healthy vision.
- Next write "My Plan" and begin to write all the steps it would take to get you to the place of your vision. Everything you would have to do to get to that place.
- Then write "My Challenges." List the things that could stand in your way and how you will deal with them to be successful.

This Week's Goals
- Next write "This Weeks Goals." Looking at your plan – what could you accomplish this week to take steps or a step toward your vision? Think of one goal you could set.

14

Even if it's one baby step. Better to focus on something that is attainable, because success will breed success. Will you: pick up a pedometer, pack a healthy lunch for work each night, sign up for an exercise class, make the doctor's appointment, get to bed earlier, or...? Pick something that you will feel good doing.

"Many calculations mean victory; few calculations mean no victory..."

~ Sun Tzu

WEEK 2

HEALTH ECONOMICS

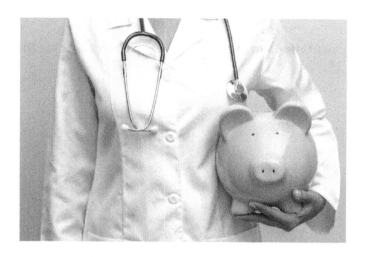

Sun Tzu clearly states the benefits of taking on smaller projects (battles) if we have to. We need to make sure battles are short and quick and familiar (physically and intellectually), so that we can rapidly produce rewards and continue the competitive endeavor or, at the very least, quickly determine whether the endeavor is worth pursuing before resources run out. This, of course, can be achieved by setting SMART goals as discussed at the end of the chapter.

Some may become confused when we discuss making battles short and quick, asking: What about long term projects - should we engage in those? The answer is yes, you can break them down into short term goals. They are connected. You can have the long term goal of walking for 30 minutes a day, but make the short term goal that you will walk for 10 minutes, up to three times a day first.

This chapter on Health Economics deals with the detrimental outcome of the increasingly high cost of chronic disease management. Through Sun Tzu's principle, it is recommended that patients adopt healthy habits and seek preventive medical care, so that medical care can be given in the earliest stages of disease – when it is a small issue and can be treated quickly. This way costly chronic-care management can be avoided. Chronic-care management is largely symptom relief, while the patients' health is perpetually being taxed and drained without adequate health promotion.

Fighting disease is very costly. But, a lot of money is spent on treating symptoms instead of the root cause of the health problem. Patients are not getting better because the focus is on treatment of symptoms, and not on prevention of disease. You can treat disease with medications, but many times that won't treat the cause, and the medications can have side effects. It's more advantageous from an economic and health standpoint to build up your health and avoid disease as much as you can.

Disease management – is a costly and unpredictable outcome that treats symptoms with drugs that can lead to side effects.

Prevention management – is a more cost-effective and predictable outcome that builds health as defense against disease.

SUN TZU said:

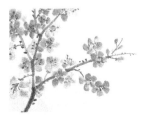

Generally, the requirements of warfare are this way: One thousand four-horse chariots, one thousand leather chariots, one hundred thousand belted armor, transporting provisions one thousand kilometers, the distribution of internal and on-the-field spending, the efforts of having guests, materials such as glue and lacquer, tributes in chariots and armor, will amount to expenses of a thousand gold pieces a day.

Only then can one hundred thousand troops be raised.

When doing battle, seek a quick victory. A long battle will blunt weapons and diminish ferocity.

If troops lay siege to a walled city, their strength will be exhausted. If the army is involved in a long campaign, the nation's resources will not suffice.

When weapons are blunted and ferocity diminished, strength exhausted and resources depleted, the neighboring rulers will take advantage of these complications.

Then even the wisest of counsels would not be able to avert the consequences that must ensue.

Therefore, I have heard of military campaigns that were clumsy but swift, but I have never seen military campaigns that were skilled but protracted. No nation has ever benefited from protracted warfare.

DR. CHAN says:

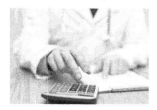

*Health wars are costly. They steal effort, money, and time - time being the most valuable. The cost will depend on the size or complexity of the battle and the duration. If it is a long health battle, there will be a huge investment of energy, money, and time that you will never get back! This is why the best health strategy is to **not** engage in a direct health battle, but instead spend your resources - time, effort, and money - in avoiding the battle altogether. That way winning will pay you – you will be healthy and have more time in a healthy state in order to enjoy your life.*

If you have to fight, make it short and quick, it keeps all costs down, monetary and otherwise.

SUN TZU said:

Therefore, if one is not fully cognizant of the dangers inherent in doing battle, one cannot fully know the benefits of doing battle.

Those skilled in doing battle do not raise troops twice, or transport provisions three times.

Take equipment from home but take provisions from the enemy. Then the army will be sufficient in both equipment and provisions.

 A nation can be impoverished by the army when it has to supply the army at great distances. When provisions are transported at great distances, the citizens will be impoverished.

DR. CHAN says:

The best strategy is to invest in your health wisely. You cannot afford costly mistakes. Competitive efforts in fighting disease do not have the predictable results that productive, preventive efforts do. It is much better to spend the efforts on something productive – PREVENTION.

Long Term Care

How do you plan for long term care costs, especially if you have chronic disease and assisted living homes are expensive? As everyone knows, Social Security is not enough to live on and Medicare is not enough to take care of medical costs.

If you spend $10,000 on well care now vs. $10,000 on sick care in the future, the money you spend now on well care will give you

*quality time. The $10,000 you spend on sick care later will not give
you quality time – it will be too late. The money on well care now is
a better return on your investment.*

Health care is an investment.

*In order to achieve your goals, you have to strategize. If you want to
save money on long-term care – spend it on well care now. Health
and wealth are two sides of the same coin (again complementary
opposites) in order to save on long term care in the future, invest in
your health now.*

SUN TZU said:

A nation can be impoverished by the army when it has to supply the
army at great distances. When provisions are transported at great
distances, the citizens will be impoverished.

Those in proximity to the army will sell goods at high prices. When
goods are expensive, the citizens' wealth will be exhausted. When
their wealth is exhausted, the peasantry will be afflicted with
increased taxes.

When all strength has been exhausted and resources depleted, all
houses in the central plains utterly impoverished, seven-tenths of the
citizens' wealth dissipated, the government's expenses from
damaged chariots, worn-out horses, armor, helmets, arrows and
crossbows, halberds and shields, draft oxen, and heavy supply
wagons, will be six-tenths of its reserves.

Therefore, a wise general will strive to feed off the enemy. One
bushel of the enemy's provisions is worth twenty of our own, one
picul of fodder is worth twenty of our own.

DR. CHAN says:

Health battles can be difficult, painful, and expensive. Not only are time, effort, and money major factors in dealing with disease, but distance is also an important factor.

The three costly factors of chronic disease management:

- ***Complex nature** – The more complex, the more expensive for all resources, e.g., multiple appointments, multiple medications, multiple procedures and surgeries.*

- ***Time** – Is the most important and the most expensive factor. You want to be healthy in order to have more quality <u>time</u>. How long will you be fighting the battle? How long will you be unhealthy? How long would you like to be able to be productive and enjoy your life?*

- ***Distance** (intellectual and physical)*
    - *Physical distance: where do you have to go to be treated?*
    - *Intellectual distance: do you have to battle the healthcare provider who doesn't believe in what you believe?*
    - *The distance to good health: small attainable goals.*

*Preventive and anti-aging medicine's mission is to give you more productive time. So you can have not only longevity, but a **healthy** long life. Invest in your health instead of disease.*

What is Preventive Healthcare?

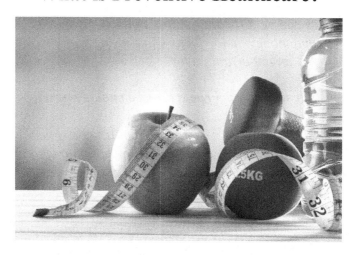

Many elderly people have chronic conditions and diseases that keep them from their normal daily activities. The vast population with chronic disease raises health insurance premiums. Learning about and practicing preventive healthcare, and maintaining good health throughout your life, is the best method to prevent disease from happening in the first place.

Preventive healthcare is planned and executed ahead of time, not when you become ill. Healthy habits are the cornerstone of preventive health, along with the conviction that building a healthy lifestyle is important, even though it requires some sacrifices.

Preventive healthcare includes: Visiting your doctor and dentist for regular check-ups and screenings, eating well, engaging in regular exercise, getting enough nightly quality sleep, having regular social connections and avoiding unhealthy substances such as: tobacco, alcohol and excessive amounts of sugar and salt.

Healthy habits are our "automatic" defense against most illnesses. They can help provide us with a long and healthy life.

Preventive healthcare staves off disease, but also finds and treats it as soon as possible. When diseases are caught early – they can be nipped in the bud and full health can be restored more quickly.

The secondary benefits of maintaining a healthy lifestyle and preventing disease is that it can help avoid a large financial loss when treating disease. Costs for preventive healthcare should be considered an investment in future health or personal insurance.

What is Age Management Medicine?

Age Management Medicine is the combination of advanced biotechnology and clinical preventive medicine. This type of medicine specializes in the early detection, prevention, treatment, as well as the reversal of age-related disorders, and diseases.

Through innovative science and research, anti-aging medicine's mission is to increase the human life span, while improving the quality of one's life as they grow older.
Harvard School of Public Health researchers found that adopting an anti-aging lifestyle in middle age can add up to 24.6 more years of productive lifespan. They found the people who enjoyed this longevity availed themselves to state-of-the-art advanced preventive care, including: preventive screenings for early disease detection, aggressive interventions, and optimal nutrition. (All of which are cornerstones of the Art of Health.)

Studies from the National Institute of Health have also proven that even the smallest changes in nutrition and fitness can increase lifespan, and help prevent disease.

SUN TZU said:

Killing the enemy is a matter of arousing anger in men; taking the enemy's wealth is a matter of reward. Therefore, in chariot battles, reward the first to capture at least ten chariots.

Replace the enemy's flags and standards with our own. Mix the captured chariots with our own and treat the captured soldiers well. This is called defeating the enemy and increasing our strength.

Therefore, the important thing in doing battle is victory, not protracted warfare.

Therefore, a general who understands warfare is the guardian of people's lives, and the ruler of the nation's security.

DR. CHAN says:

Don't just beat disease – be victorious, be healthy. Generate benefits from your efforts, and make winning your health be your payment.

You have choices for your future: In the next ten years if you are battling a disease – you will gain nothing but bills, side effects, fatigue, etc.

In the next ten years if you focus on your health - you will gain quality of life and longevity.

Medications may add years to your life, but they may not add life to your years!

Wellness Warrior Actions: Week 2

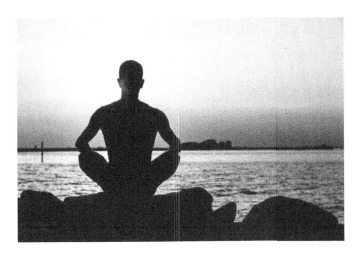

Vision meditation

- Have your journal ready to record your thoughts after you meditate.
- Sit in a private, quiet, and comfortable place.
- Close your eyes and relax.
- Take a deep breath in and exhale three times to empty the air in your chest (this will start your deep breathing).
- Take a breath for each number as you count backwards from 10 to 1, as you relax your body and center yourself. Notice where there is tension and let it go with your breath.
- Think about how your week went. How did you do on last week's goal or goals?
- Is there anything you could have done differently?
- For week **2** - Think about the resources you could use towards your health to insure a healthy future. Where could you spend the time, money, and effort to be healthier?
- Refer back to your healthy vision. Begin to see who you would like to be in the future, a few months from now, a year from now, 10 years from now. See yourself as very healthy. What does that look like? What does that feel like?

Journaling

- Write "Week 2" in your journal and record what you accomplished this week in keeping your goal or goals. Write any observations you may have and what you may want to do differently.

This week's goals

- Write what resources you are using to be healthier in the future? Where are you investing your time, effort, and money? What changes could you make for the future? What is a health issue you are having? What small step could you take this week to address the issue? Set it up as a SMART goal.

- To help achieve your goals, make sure they are SMART goals:

  S – Specific: What exactly do you want to do? Clearly define your goal.
  M – Measurable: How can you measure and track progress?
  A – Attainable: Can you achieve it in the time frame?
  R – Relevant: Is it relevant to your long-term goals?
  T – Time bound: When will you take action? Time sensitive goals are more likely to be achieved than a loose thought of action without an end time attached to it.

"When doing battle seek a quick victory."

~ Sun Tzu

WEEK 3

PLANNING THE ATTACK: UNITY AND FOCUS

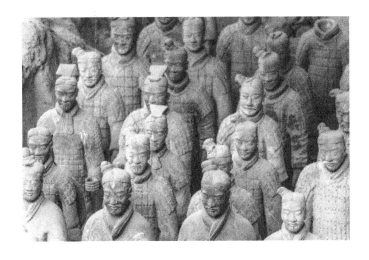

The best leader is not the one who fights 100 battles and wins 100 battles, it is the one who has no battles; who does not fight. Even if you win the battle, you've lost the war.

Sun Tzu teaches that unity and focus are the strength of an organization. The goal of unity and focus is to win without conflict. In health this is to be healthy and free of chronic disease, so you don't have to battle disease.

Sun Tzu lists the basic forms of attack with the worst being to directly attack when the opponent's position is strong, or when a disease is strongly attacking you. The best advantage is to use small focused steps.

The five areas of knowledge will be covered in this chapter. These areas determine our ability to unify and focus.

SUN TZU said:

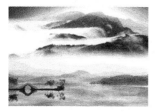

Generally in warfare, keeping a nation intact is best, destroying a nation second best;

Keeping an army intact is best, destroying an army second best;

Keeping a battalion intact is best, destroying a battalion second best;

Keeping a company intact is best, destroying a company second best;

Keeping a squad intact is best, destroying a squad second best.

Therefore, to achieve a hundred victories in a hundred battles is not the highest excellence; to subjugate the enemy's army without doing battle is the highest of excellence.

DR. CHAN says:

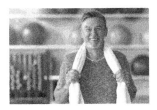

If you have unity, you are whole and strong. It is a unity of all of the parts of the body, working in harmony – holistically. If not, you are broken or sick.

Focus means winning by intelligence; to thwart a battle by intelligent planning. The leaders and heroes are the teachers and preventers.

The goal is to be so healthy that disease cannot challenge you. There will be no need to do battle. To achieve optimal health – you must focus on prevention.

SUN TZU said:

Therefore, the best warfare strategy is to attack the enemy's plans, next is to attack alliances, next is to attack the army, and the worst is to attack a walled city.

Laying siege to a city is only done when other options are not available.

To build protective shields, armored wagons, and make ready other arms and equipment will require at least three months.
To build earthen mounds against the walls will require another three months.

If the general cannot control his temper and sends troops to swarm the walls, one third of them will be killed, and the city will still not be taken. This is the kind of calamity when laying siege to a walled city.

Therefore, one who is skilled in warfare principles subdues the enemy without doing battle, takes the enemy's walled city without attacking, and overthrows the enemy quickly, without protracted warfare.

DR. CHAN says:

The best doctor is not the one who fights against disease and wins all the time, but rather, it is <u>the one who wins without fighting.</u>

Television dramas and media stories like to depict doctors as lifesaving heroes. But, the doctor who is the true hero, is the one preventing disease before it starts.

Our society is going through a paradigm shift and people are realizing the benefits of choosing health care instead of sick care.

The best health strategy is to attack disease's plans and infiltrations by engaging in preventive medicine and living a healthy lifestyle. If you have not been doing that, then sooner rather than later, you will have to battle against the disease's army and walled city.

The best way to attack is to change your belief system to: health care vs. sick care.

Change your mindset first:
- *Frequency is more important that intensity.*
- *Focus on small steps rather than big steps.*
- *Growth comes from focus over time.*

If you are driving a car and turn the steering wheel just a few degrees to the right or left – you will eventually end up in a very different place. You want to make a series of small successes to get you where you want to be.

To begin to build your protective health, arm yourself with the tools of a healthy immune system. Becoming adept in the Art of Health will require around 12 weeks.

If you do not arm yourself with health and healthy tools, you will find it will take many more months to battle illness and as we discussed before, it will also take resources and effort, and it may be that then, it will be a battle that you cannot win.

SUN TZU said:

His aim must be to take All-Under-Heaven intact.

Therefore, weapons will not be blunted, and gains will be intact.

These are the principles of planning attacks.

Generally in warfare:

If ten times the enemy's strength, surround them;

If five times, attack them;

If double, divide them;

If equal, be able to fight them;

If fewer, be able to evade them;

If weaker, be able to avoid them.

Therefore, a smaller army that is inflexible will be captured by a larger one.

A general is the safeguard of the nation. When this support is in place, the nation will be strong. When this support is not in place, the nation will not be strong.

There are three ways the ruler can bring difficulty to the army:

1) To order an advance when not realizing the army is in no position to advance, or to order a withdrawal when not realizing the army is

in no position to withdraw. This is called entangling the army.

2) By not knowing the army's matters, and administering the army the same as administering civil matters, the officers and troops will be confused.

3) By not knowing the army's calculations, and taking command of the army, the officers and troops will be hesitant.

DR. CHAN says:

To keep your gains (e.g., health, time, money, and energy) intact, you must plan how you attack the potential of disease.

Of course you want to be ten times stronger than disease and surround it automatically with a healthy immune system. To stay ten times stronger than disease you must stay vigilant in your quest to be the healthiest you can be.

If you are five times stronger, you can still attack with strong medicine.

If you cannot bombard disease, then do what you need to do first. Divide your symptoms and deal with them one at a time.

If you are weak, then build yourself up first and avoid direct confrontation with disease whenever possible.

You and your healthcare providers are the safeguard of your health. When good support is in place, you will be strong and healthy, when it's not in place, you will be sick, or on the verge of sickness.

You can disrupt unity and bring difficulty on yourself by self-sabotage. The enemy can be you.

There are three ways you can bring illness on yourself:

1) *By asking too much or too little of your body. By not realizing you are in no position to expend the energy needed to perform certain tasks, or not realizing you should be using your body more.*

2) *By not seeing your healthcare providers and not educating yourself on general health matters to learn what is best for your health.*

3) *By not knowing your health details and calculations (e.g., lab results, blood pressure, glucose levels, cholesterol, nutrition evaluation, weight, etc.) so you can adjust your lifestyle to improve or maintain your health.*

Lifestyle changes are better than diabetes drugs

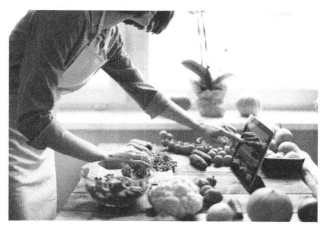

Type 2 diabetes is an epidemic in the United States. According to the Centers for Disease Control, the number of Americans with diabetes could triple by the year 2050. Currently, one in 10 U.S. adults has the disease, but if it continues to progress, it could grow to one in three. And the numbers are sky rocketing in children and teens.

Diabetes is a serious chronic disease that is responsible for about $170 billion in health care costs. The disease presents serious health complications, including increased risk of cardiovascular disease, kidney disease, nerve damage, blindness, foot damage, skin conditions, Alzheimer's disease, and other conditions and complications.

One of the oldest diabetes drugs works better than the newer drugs, according to researchers at Johns Hopkins School of Medicine. They compared metformin, which the FDA approved more than 15 years ago and is now available in a cheap generic form, with several newer drugs. Metformin proved to be as good as, or better, than the other drugs, and had fewer side effects. Some of the newer drugs had serious side effects.

This is not to highlight metformin, but to state that there is a therapy older than this drug that's the most effective at preventing and controlling diabetes, and has no adverse side effects. It's *called – a <u>healthy lifestyle</u>, which includes a healthy diet and exercise.*

It was first proven and published in 2002, in the New England Journal of Medicine, that lifestyle changes are twice as effective as metformin. The findings were a result of a multi-year Diabetes Prevention Program. This was left out of the current reporting of the Johns Hopkins study and, in my opinion, a serious omission. The first treatment recommendation for Type 2 Diabetes that should be made, is the best one of all - healthy lifestyle modifications.

SUN TZU said:

When the army is confused and hesitant, the neighboring rulers will take advantage. This is called a confused and hesitant army leading another to victory.

Therefore, there are five factors of knowledge when in competition:

1) One who knows when he can fight, and when he cannot fight;

2) One who knows how to use both large and small forces;

3) One who knows how to unite upper and lower ranks in purpose;

4) One who is prepared and waits for the unprepared;

5) One whose general is able and who can act with no interference by a ruler.

These five factors are the way to know who will win.

Therefore I say: One who knows the enemy and knows himself will not be in danger in a hundred battles.

One who does not know the enemy but knows himself will sometimes win, sometimes lose. One who does not know the enemy and does not know himself will be in danger in every battle.

DR. CHAN says:

When your body is confused or hesitant, it opens the door to potential disease taking advantage.

You must know five things in order to win against disease:

1) **You must know when you can avoid battle, and when you must attack.** *This depends on how strong you are and how strong the disease is. How do you know how strong you are? It is relative to disease. SUN TZU said to compare. (Use the 5 Elements in the first chapter to assess your strategic position.) If you are sick, the 5 Elements model can be used to compare yourself against disease. If you are well, you can use the 5 Elements model to compare yourself against your future self – who you want to become.*

2) **You must know when to use both large and small forces against disease.** *Large forces would be surgery, powerful medicines and antibiotics. Small forces would be natural and gentle medicines.*

3) **You must know how to unite your healthcare support in a common purpose.** *Develop your preventive health plan with your trusted healthcare providers.*

4) **You must know how to be prepared for the unexpected.** *Always build up your resilience to prepare for unexpected health events.*

5) *You must have capable healthcare providers who practice state-of-the-art preventive medicine without interference from outside sources.* *You may need to recruit health professionals who practice "above and beyond" the standard of care.*

Focus on Prevention – If you don't have to fight, you're more likely to win.

Wellness Warrior Actions: Week 3

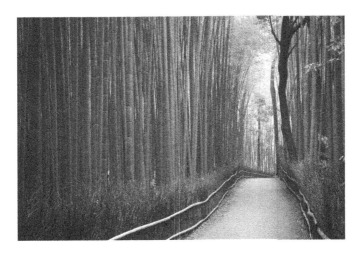

Vision meditation
- Have your journal ready to record your thoughts after you meditate.
- Sit in a private, quiet, and comfortable place.
- Close your eyes and relax.
- Take a deep breath in and exhale three times to empty the air in your chest (this will start your deep breathing).
- Take a breath for each number as you count backwards from 10 to 1, as you relax your body and center yourself. Notice where there is tension and let it go with your breath.
- Think about how your week went. How did you do on the past week's goal or goals?

- Is there anything you would have done differently?
- **For week 3** – Meditate on your Unity and Focus. Are you focusing on prevention? Do you have your healthcare providers unified to focus on prevention? Know yourself – what do you need to do to arm yourself preventively?
- Refer back to your healthy vision. Begin to see what it would look like in the future if you took those actions and armed yourself preventively. What would that look like a few months from now, a year from now, 10 years from now? See yourself as very healthy. What does that look like? What does that feel like?

Journaling:

- Write "Week 3" in your journal and record what you accomplished this week in keeping your goal or goals. Write any observations you may have and what you may want to do differently.

- **This week's goals**
  How are you unified and focused on your preventive health? What changes do you need to make for the future? What small step could you take this week to address the issue? Write it down as a SMART goal.

- To help achieve your goals, make sure they are SMART goals:
  S – Specific: What exactly do you want to do? Clearly define your goal.
  M – Measurable: How can you measure and track progress?
  A – Attainable: Can you achieve it in the time frame?
  R – Relevant: Is it relevant to your long-term goals?
  T – Time bound: When will you take action? Time sensitive goals are more likely to be achieved than a loose thought of action without an end time attached to it.

"Therefore those who win every battle are not really skillful – those who render others' armies helpless without fighting are the best of all."

~Sun Tzu

WEEK 4

HEALTH POSITIONING

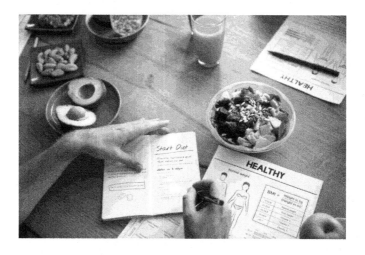

Health positioning is positioning yourself for future health and wellness. You must first and always defend and protect yourself against disease, but also build yourself up before taking medication. Defend your current good health and attack disease at the first sign – when you are strong and have the resources. We must maintain a defensive mindset and invest in our health now, knowing that it will be much more costly to treat illness.

SUN TZU said:

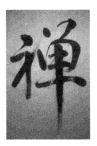

In ancient times, those skilled in warfare made themselves invincible and then waited for the enemy to become vulnerable. Being invincible depends on one self, but the enemy's vulnerability depends on himself.

Those skilled in warfare can make themselves invincible, but cannot necessarily cause the enemy to be vulnerable. Therefore it is said one may know how to win but cannot necessarily do it.

One takes on invincibility defending; one takes on vulnerability attacking.

One takes on sufficiency defending, one takes on deficiency attacking."

Those skilled in defense conceal themselves in the lowest depths of the Earth. Those skilled in attack move in the highest reaches of the Heavens. Therefore, they are able to protect themselves and achieve complete victory.

DR. CHAN says:

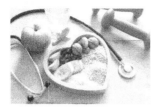

In health, as in all things, you must position your mind to do your best. Life is a competition from the beginning. At the point of conception – 300 million sperm are competing to fertilize one egg. Only one will win, and begin to form ...you. Why would you not love yourself, do your best, and defend your health?

There is a fundamental lie that people tell themselves, it is that they are not enough. This is self-sabotage. People try to protect themselves and cover the deficit they feel, but trying superficial ways to boost their confidence will not work. You must expose the lie, be honest, acknowledge your fears and show your vulnerability. Be authentic, so you can love and protect yourself and have optimal wellbeing.

SUN TZU said:

Perceiving a victory when it is perceived by all is not the highest excellence.

Winning battles such that the whole world cries 'Excellent!' is not the highest excellence.

For lifting an autumn down is not considered great strength, seeing the sun and the moon is not considered a sign of sharp vision, hearing thunder is not considered a sign of sensitive hearing.

In ancient times, those who were skilled in warfare gained victory where victory was easily gained.

Therefore, the victories from those skilled in warfare are not considered of great wisdom or courage, because their victories have no complications.

No miscalculations mean the victories are certain, achieving victory over those who have already lost.

Therefore, those skilled in warfare establish positions that make them invincible and do not miss opportunities to attack the enemy.

Therefore, a victorious army first obtains conditions for victory, then seeks to do battle. A defeated army first seeks to do battle, then obtains conditions for victory.

DR. CHAN says:

This is the basis of my philosophy of medicine:

A winning mindset creates winning situations. Build your health before you attack disease or take medications. Medications can have side-effects and many medications cause nutrition deficiencies. Meditate before you medicate.

Those who are unwise don't build themselves up. They allow themselves to get sick, then take medications, hoping they get better.

Most people go to their doctors when they are sick. You should really go to your doctor so you don't get sick.

If you are weak – build your foundation; do not fight until you are strong. Focus on building your strength and health.

Engage in small battles that you can win, that are easy. Good defense allows you to pick your battles and win.

Great physicians are not those who focus primarily on healing the few sickest patients, and derive fame and glory from curing them.

The great physicians are those who help the sick as well as the healthy patients become even healthier, so they are able to achieve optimal health.

Weight Management and Health

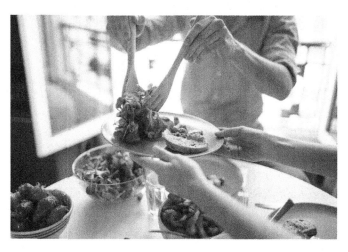

A healthy weight is important for overall health, therefore, it is a good place to start to build a healthy foundation. It can help you prevent and control many diseases and conditions. If you are overweight, you are at a higher risk of developing serious health problems, including heart disease, high blood pressure, type 2 diabetes, and cancer. Maintaining a healthy weight not only helps you lower your risk for developing health problems, but also helps you feel good about yourself, and gives you the energy you need to enjoy life.

Being Mindful - for weight management and health

When you are mindful about choosing and eating food, you will begin to make better choices and naturally want the foods that are good for your body.

When you are relaxed and mindful when eating, you digest nutrients better and get more out of the food you eat, as well as eliminate toxins more efficiently. You will begin to notice the foods that make you feel good and give you better energy. You will naturally begin to want those foods that are good for you.

When you are relaxed and mindful in your life, you will begin to eat the right foods for the right reasons. You will not eat because you are tired, bored, upset, or nervous. You will eat to nourish and give your body the fuel it needs, and then you will address other issues in mindful ways.

When you are mindful, you will begin to choose those things that are good for you, as an individual. For example, you will choose the right exercise for you because it is one you enjoy, that makes you feel good.

Take advantage of the power of the moment.

SUN TZU said:

Those skilled in warfare cultivate the Way, and preserve the Law, therefore, they govern victory and defeat.

The factors in warfare are: First, measurement; second, quantity; third, calculation; fourth, comparison; and fifth, victory.

Measurements are derived from Ground, quantities are derived from measurement, calculations are derived from quantities, comparisons are derived from calculations, and victories are derived from comparisons.

A victorious army is like a ton against an ounce; a defeated army is like an ounce against a ton! The victorious army is like pent up waters released, bursting through a deep gorge. This is formation.

DR. CHAN says:

Those who are healthy make a plan and cultivate habits. Victories are derived when you position yourself and become healthier, keeping disease at bay. The factors of your health positioning are:
- *The Measurement and Quantities of your physical being – age, height, weight, BMI, blood pressure, lab scores, test results, food measurements.*
- *The Calculations – evaluate your health and habits at this point, which includes calculating the cost of health now and in the future.*
- *Comparisons – to others and to your past and future self. How much healthier are you than a few years ago?*

Wellness Warrior Actions: Week 4

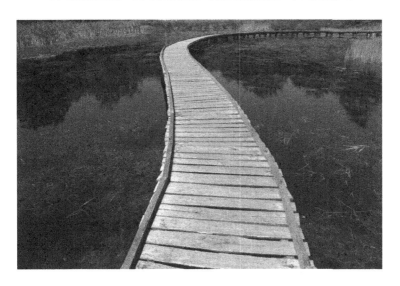

Vision meditation

- Have your journal ready to record your thoughts after you meditate.
- Sit in a private, quiet, and comfortable place.
- Close your eyes and relax.
- Take a deep breath in and exhale three times to empty the air in your chest (this will start your deep breathing).
- Take a breath for each number and count backwards from 10 to 1, as you relax your body and center yourself. Notice where there is tension and let it go with your breath.
- Think about how your week went. How did you do on the past week's goal or goals?
- Is there anything you would have done differently?
- **For week 4** – Meditate on your Health Positioning. Are you in a strong health position? Are your healthcare providers helping you to build your strength? Are you building your strength for a healthy future?
- Refer back to your healthy vision. Begin to see what it would look like in the future if you took action to build a strong health position. What would that look like a few

months from now, a year from now, 10 years from now? See yourself as very healthy. What does that look like? What does that feel like?

Journaling:

- Write "Week 4" in your journal and record what you accomplished this week in keeping your goal or goals. Write any observations you may have and what you may want to do differently.

This week's goals:

Is your health position strong? Look at your Measurements and Quantities – what do you need to work on to have stronger health? Calculations – what habit could you incorporate in your daily life to be stronger in the future? What investment could you make to ensure a stronger health position? How do you compare to your old self and your future self? What changes do you need to make to be stronger in the future? What small step or steps could you take this week for your future health positioning?
Write it down as a SMART goal.

S – Specific: What exactly do you want to do? Clearly define your goal.
M – Measurable: How can you measure and track progress?
A – Attainable: Can you achieve it in the time frame?
R – Relevant: Is it relevant to your long-term goals?
T – Time bound: When will you take action? Time sensitive goals are more likely to be achieved than a loose thought of action without an end time attached to it.

"Those who are healthy make a plan and cultivate habits."

~ Dr. Kevin Chan

WEEK 5

INNOVATIVE HEALTHCARE

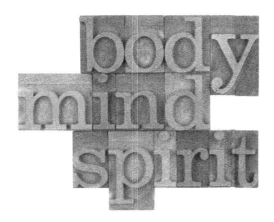

Sun Tzu titled this chapter "Force," but the translation means something akin to momentum - the blending of standard strategies and new strategies in order to win. We will interpret this as "innovation." In health care, the standard strategy is conventional medicine and the new strategy is integrative medicine. Anything you do in life requires innovation if you want to be successful; so it is in healthcare. Start with conventional medicine to engage, but use integrative medicine to innovate, to gain momentum, and achieve victory – optimal health.

SUN TZU said:

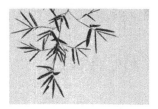

Generally, commanding many is like commanding a few. It is a matter of dividing them into groups. Doing battle with a large army is like doing battle with a small army. It is a matter of communications through flags and pennants.

Due to common and uncommon maneuvers, an army can withstand the enemy's attack and not be defeated.

The army will be like throwing a stone against an egg; it is a matter of weakness and strength.

Generally, in battle, use the common to engage the enemy and the uncommon to gain victory. Those skilled at uncommon maneuvers are as endless as the heavens and earth, and as inexhaustible as the rivers and seas.

DR. CHAN says:

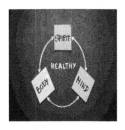

You always want to pick small battles so you can win. Win the small health battles, so they don't become large health battles. Those who engage in conventional medicine and then use uncommon strategies, through integrative medicine, will have uncommon victories and health.

Innovation, or uncommon methods, also includes the element of surprise, which when used timely at specific situations, will generate even better health outcomes. For example, when you are stuck or have plateaued in an exercise program, do something surprisingly different to gain momentum and move forward.

SUN TZU said:

Like the sun and the moon, they set and rise again. Like the four seasons, they end and begin again. There are no more than five musical notes, yet the variations in the five notes cannot all be heard. There are no more than five basic colors, yet the variations in the five colors cannot all be seen. There are no more than five basic flavors, yet the variations in the five flavors cannot all be tasted.

In battle, there are no more than two types of attacks: Common and uncommon, yet the variations of the common and uncommon cannot all be anticipated.

The common and the uncommon produce each other, like an endless circle. Who can comprehend them?

The rush of torrential waters tossing boulders illustrates force. The strike of a bird of prey breaking the body of its target illustrates timing.

Therefore, the force of those skilled in warfare is overwhelming and their timing precise.

Their force is like a drawn crossbow and their timing is like the release of the trigger.

Even in the midst of the turbulence of battle, the fighting seemingly chaotic, they are not confused. Even in the midst of the turmoil of battle, the troops seemingly going around in circles, they cannot be defeated.

51

DR. CHAN says:

In healthcare there are two types of attacks: common and uncommon, or conventional and integrative medicine. They produce each other and offer a variety of strategies and attacks. Use the common to get what you want and the uncommon to win. Innovate from something old. The force of the two is what's needed to defeat disease. I practice strategic integrative medicine, so I can offer my patients more options to do "whatever it takes" to get and stay healthy.

If you are doing battle with health issues, you will be in control and have more options for success if your timing is right.

Your use of timeliness is key to success. Be mindful of speed and quickness when employing innovative techniques. Speed is how fast you are moving in your current direction (don't wait, you have to move forward). Quickness is how fast you can change direction – the ability to change quickly if you find you are moving in the wrong direction.

Strategic Integrative Medicine

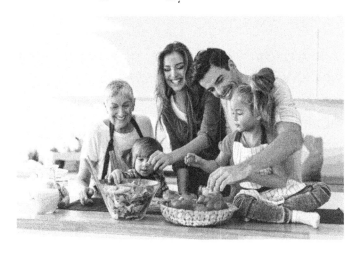

Strategic Integrative Medicine is a progressive style of medicine that incorporates the best practices of integrative, functional, and mind-body medicine in the framework of Sun Tzu's strategic system with the scientific application of ancient metaphysical principles.

Integrative Medicine combines alternative medicine and therapies with conventional medicine to diagnose and treat disease. It focuses on prevention rather than treating disease, and also promotes a strong patient-physician relationship.

Functional Medicine is a form of integrative medicine that uses a systems approach to address the root causes of ill health and disease, many times in its preventive stage. It focuses on the interactions of the body's systems with the environment and with each other. Through biochemical diagnostic testing, to evaluate how systems are functioning, functional medicine discovers and treats the underlying causes of disease and imbalances.

The Seven Pillars of Integrative and Functional Medicine:

Healthy Lifestyle (Nutrition, Exercise, Stress Management)
Hormonal and Neurotransmitter Health
Cardiovascular Health
Gastrointestinal Health
Detoxification and Biotransformation Health
Neurological and Mitochondria (energy production) Health
Immune Health and Reduction of Inflammation

Mind-Body Medicine (META-Medicine) is based on the science of the bio-psycho-social connection. It is based on scientific evidence emerging from more than 30 years of brain scans and research that there is a body-mind-social connection that affects health.

META-Medicine focuses on how specific stress triggers, emotions, and beliefs affect specific organ symptoms and disease. It helps healthcare professionals and their patients understand how stressors, thoughts, feelings, and behaviors affect health and personal development. It also explains the specific points and phases of the healing process. META-Medicine professionals practice META-Health, which incorporates specific lifestyle prescriptions of integrative medicine, as well as conventional medicine, to be more effective in helping their patients.

- *META-Health is the connection between the bio-psycho-social framework and the art of self-healing.*
- *To be META-Healthy means you are aware of your body's intelligence, stress triggers, emotions and beliefs that affect your body, and take conscious action towards self-healing.*
- *META-Healing is the transformation process to achieve body-mind-social or META-Health, and is based on mind-body techniques.*

SUN TZU said:

Disorder came from order, fear came from courage, weakness came from strength.

Disorder coming from order is a matter of organization; fear coming from courage is a matter of force, weakness coming from strength is a matter of formation.

Therefore, those skilled in moving the enemy use formation that makes the enemy respond.

They offer bait that which the enemy must take, manipulating the enemy to move while they wait in ambush.

Those skilled in warfare seek victory through force and do not require too much from individuals. Therefore, they are able to select the right men and exploit force.

One who exploits force commands men into battle like rolling logs and boulders. Logs and boulders are still when on flat ground, but roll when on steep ground. Square shapes are still, but round shapes roll.

Therefore, those skilled in warfare use force by making the troops in battle like boulders rolling down a steep mountain. This is force.

DR. CHAN says:

Through complementary opposite philosophy, you can turn disease into health, and chaos into order. But first you have to be skilled in the formation of health and battling disease. Those who are skilled will choose the right health care providers to help create the force needed to innovate their health care.

Wellness Warrior Actions: Week 5

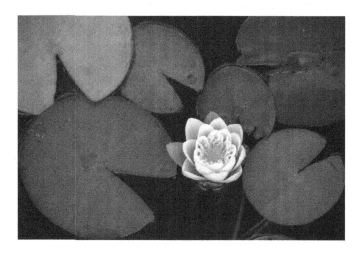

Vision meditation

- Have your journal ready to record your thoughts after you meditate.
- Sit in a private, quiet, and comfortable place.
- Close your eyes and relax.
- Take a deep breath in and exhale three times to empty the air in your chest (this will start your deep breathing).
- Take a breath for each number and count backwards from 10 to 1, as you relax your body and center yourself. Notice where there is tension and let it go with your breath.
- Think about how your week went. How did you do on the past week's goal or goals?
- Is there anything you would have done differently?
- **For week 5** – Meditate on how you could innovate your health care. What could you do that is innovative and integrative? Read through the Seven Pillars of Integrative Medicine again – what area do you need to pursue, or could you pursue, to help you become a wellness warrior?
- Refer back to your healthy vision. Begin to see what it would look like in the future if you took action to innovate your health care. What would that look like a few months from now, a year from now, 10 years from now? See

56

yourself as very healthy. What does that look like? What does that feel like?

Journaling:

- Write "Week 5" in your journal and record what you accomplished this week in keeping your goal or goals. Write any observations you may have and what you may want to do differently.

This week's goals:

In what area of the Seven Pillars of Integrative Medicine could you use innovative health care? What do you need to do to make that happen? Research an integrative healthcare provider? Call and make an appointment for a consultation? What step or steps could you take this week to make new changes or introduce innovative new methods to your healthcare? Write it down as a SMART goal.

S – Specific: What exactly do you want to do? Clearly define your goal.

M – Measurable: How can you measure and track progress?

A – Attainable: Can you achieve it in the time frame?

R – Relevant: Is it relevant to your long-term goals?

T – Time bound: When will you take action? Time sensitive goals are more likely to be achieved than a loose thought of action without an end time attached to it.

"Generally, in battle, use the common to engage the enemy and the uncommon to gain victory. Those skilled at uncommon maneuvers are as endless as the heavens and earth, and as inexhaustible as the rivers and seas."

~ Sun Tzu

WEEK 6

WEAKNESS AND STRENGTH IN

HEALTH

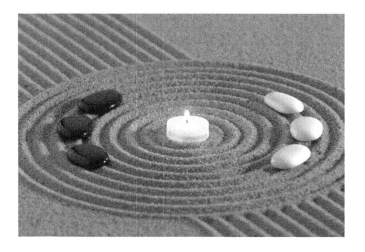

Sun Tzu teaches that through the complementary opposites of weakness and strength we are able to turn challenges into opportunities. The yin and yang of healthcare: if extreme in one area, it gives rise to the opposite. (Yin is only yin when compared to yang. Yang is only yang when compared to yin.)

Sun Tzu compares knowledge and ignorance with strength and weakness. He encourages focusing strengths on the weakness of the opposition, so you can exploit the opposition. In relation to your healthcare – stay focused and know your strengths and weaknesses. Use your strengths by bringing in experts to attack any weaknesses in your health.

SUN TZU said:

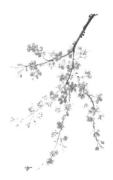

Generally the one who first occupies the battlefield awaiting the enemy is at ease; the one who comes later and rushes into battle is fatigued.

Therefore those skilled at warfare move the enemy, and are not moved by the enemy.

Getting the enemy to approach on his own accord is a matter of showing him advantage; stopping him from approaching is a matter of showing him harm.

Therefore, if the enemy is at ease, be able to exhaust him; if the enemy is well fed, be able to starve him; if the enemy is settled, be able to move him; appear at places where he must rush to defend, and rush to places where he least expects.

DR. CHAN says:

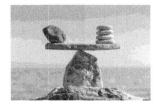

The patient who has worked on their health and is ready to attack any sign of disease, is at ease. The patient who has not worked on their health and rushes to do battle with disease, is already fatigued.

Those who are skilled at health have an advantage against disease – they know how to starve it, exhaust it and defend in places it does not expect.

Therefore, get healthy to exhaust disease in its early stages, do not offer anything it can feed on or help it to settle in, do the unexpected and use integrative protocols to catch disease at its weakest.

SUN TZU said:

To march over a thousand kilometers without becoming distressed, march over where the enemy is not present.

To be certain to take what you attack, attack where the enemy cannot defend.

To be certain of safety when defending, defend where the enemy cannot attack.

Therefore, against those skilled in attack, the enemy does not know where to defend.

Against those skilled in defense, the enemy does not know where to attack.
Subtle, subtle; they become formless. Mysterious, mysterious; they

become soundless. Therefore, they are the masters of the enemy's fate.

DR. CHAN says:

In order to be healthy and not become distressed, become healthy when disease is not present. This way you can attack disease early and be certain of defending yourself.

If you become healthy and skilled at defense and attack, disease will not know where to defend or attack.

Be mindful as you make healthy choices; take daily steps to adopt healthy habits and you will quietly become master of your health.

SUN TZU said:

To achieve an advance that cannot be hampered, rush to his weak points. To achieve a withdrawal that cannot be pursued, depart with superior speed.

Therefore, if we want to do battle, even if the enemy is protected by high walls and deep moats, he cannot but do battle, because we attack what he must rescue. If we do not want to do battle, even if we merely draw a line on the ground, he will not do battle, because we divert his movements.

Therefore, if we can make the enemy show his position while we are formless, the enemy is divided while we are at full force.

If our army is at full force and the enemy is divided, then we will attack him at ten times his strength.

Therefore, we are many and the enemy few. If we attack our many against his few, the enemy will be in dire straits.

The place of battle must not be made known to the enemy. If it is not known, then the enemy must prepare to defend many places.

If the enemy prepares to defend many places, then his forces will be few in number.

Therefore, if the enemy prepares to defend the front, the back will be weak. If he prepares to defend the back, the front will be weak. If he prepares to defend the left, the right will be weak. If he prepares to defend the right, the left will be weak. If he prepares to defend everywhere, everywhere will be weak.

The few are those preparing to defend against others, the many are those who make others prepare to defend against them.

Therefore, if one knows the place of battle and the day of battle, he can march a thousand kilometers and do battle.

If one does not know the place of battle and the day of battle, then his left cannot aid his right, his right cannot aid his left, his front cannot aid his back, and his back cannot aid his front.

How much less so if he is separated by tens of kilometers, or even a few kilometers.

Though Yueh's troops were many, what advantage was this to them? You can achieve victory.

Though the enemy is many, he can be prevented from doing battle. Therefore, know the enemy's plans and calculate his strengths and weaknesses.

Provoke him, to know his patterns of movement.

Determine his position, to know the ground of death and of life. Probe him, to know where he is strong and where he is weak.

DR. CHAN says:

*Know your strengths and weaknesses and have a strategy **for** health and **against** disease. Know diseases strengths and weaknesses. Even if disease is strong, strategy and positioning are very powerful when planning your defense or attack.*

Stay focused and do not spread yourself too thin. Less is more. Take small steps.

Use the 80/20 Rule (also known as the Pareto Principle), which states that roughly 80% of the effects from events come from 20% of the causes. Address the 20% of the actions for your health that will bring 80% of the results you want.

The 80/20 Rule

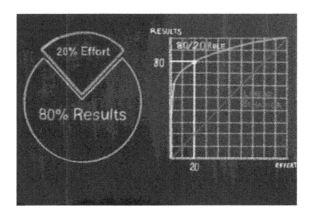

The 80/20 rule, or the Pareto Principle, is a common theory in business and economics. The concept was first introduced by Vilfredo Federico Damaso Pareto, who was an Italian philosopher and economist. He published a paper in 1896 on uneven distribution, whereby he noted that 80% of the land in Italy was owned by 20% of the population. He first noticed this phenomenon when 20% of the pea plants in his garden generated 80% of the

healthy pea pods. This caused him to study the principle of uneven distribution and he investigated different industries. He found that 80% of the production of goods typically came from just 20% of the companies. The principle was further studied and verified that: 80% of results will come from 20% of the actions.

SUN TZU said:

The ultimate skill is to take up a position where you are formless.

If you are formless, the most penetrating spies will not be able to discern you, or the wisest counsels will not be able to do calculations against you.

With formation, the army achieves victories yet they do not understand how. Everyone knows the formation by which you achieved victory, yet no one knows the formations by which you were able to create victory.

Therefore, your strategy for victories in battle is not repetitious, and your formations in response to the enemy are endless.

The army's formation is like water. The water's formation avoids the high and rushes to the low.

So an army's formation avoids the strong and rushes to the weak. Water's formation adapts to the ground when flowing. So then an army's formation adapts to the enemy to achieve victory.

Therefore, an army does not have constant force or have constant formation. Those who are able to adapt and change in accord with the enemy and achieve victory are called divine.

Therefore, of the five elements, none a constant victor; of the four seasons, none has constant position; the sun has short and long spans, and the moon waxes and wanes.

DR. CHAN says:

Be formless in your health care - like water, and the five elements, and the four seasons, and the sun and the moon - so your responses to disease can be adaptable and limitless. Change your health strategies in accordance with your symptoms.

Do not rush to the highs, but to the lows, meaning quickly take care of the small health issues, so they don't turn into large health issues. Avoid the strong by rushing to the weak or small areas of disease, so they don't become strong.

Those who are able to adapt and change in their health care are wellness warriors and can achieve optimal health.

Wellness Warrior Actions: Week 6

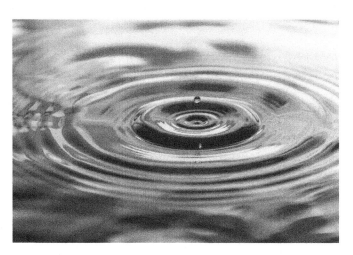

Vision Meditation

- Have your journal ready to record your thoughts after you meditate.
- Sit in a private, quiet, and comfortable place.
- Close your eyes and relax.
- Take a deep breath in and exhale three times to empty the air in your chest (this will start your deep breathing).
- Take a breath for each number and count backwards from 10 to 1, as you relax your body and center yourself. Notice where there is tension and let it go with your breath.
- Think about how your week went. How did you do on the past week's goal or goals?
- Is there anything you would have done differently?
- **For week 6** – Meditate on the strengths and weaknesses of your health and in your health care. See your weaknesses as opportunities. See yourself as water – being very adaptable and becoming healthier.
- Refer back to your healthy vision. Begin to see what it would look like in the future if you took action and used your strengths to make weaknesses health opportunities. What would that look like a few months from now, a year

from now, 10 years from now? See yourself as very healthy. What does that look like? What does that feel like?

Journaling:

- Write "Week 6" in your journal and record what you accomplished this week in keeping your goal or goals. Write any observations you may have and what you may want to do differently in the future.

This week's goals:

- Write down your strengths and weaknesses in health and in health care. Following the 80/20 Rule, what are the few goals (the 20%) that you could take action on, that would give you 80% of the results that you want? Is it to find the right healthcare provider, develop an eating plan or exercise plan? Make sure they are SMART goals.

    S – Specific: What exactly do you want to do? Clearly define your goal.
    M – Measurable: How can you measure and track progress?
    A – Attainable: Can you achieve it in the time frame?
    R – Relevant: Is it relevant to your long-term goals?
    T – Time bound: When will you take action? Time sensitive goals are more likely to be achieved than a loose thought of action without an end time attached to it.

"Know your strengths and weaknesses and have a strategy for health and against disease."

~ Dr. Kevin Chan

WEEK 7

DIRECT CONFRONTATION AND
ADAPTABILITY IN HEALTH

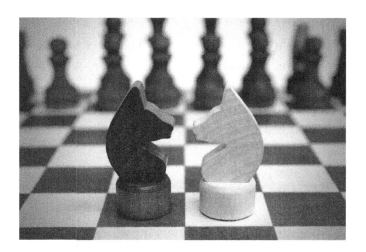

1. Direct Confrontation

Sun Tzu teaches that confrontation is not the best strategy to success. We should always prepare for confrontation, but try and avoid it. In this chapter Sun Tzu reminds us of the disasters that can take place when one rushes to confrontation without preparing. When confrontation is unavoidable, use good communication and shared vision as main strategies. Also use good timing and control emotions to avoid mistakes.

In healthcare, confrontation of a disease is not the best strategy. You should always prepare for such a confrontation, but avoid it and prepare for conflict by living a healthy lifestyle and catching any disease in its earliest stages. Also, by seeing your healthcare providers regularly and having preventive testing done. Use good communication with your doctors and maintain a vision of your strategies for a healthy future. Use good timing when scheduling health appointments, as not making preventive appointments, labs, and screenings can be a mistake you don't want to make.

Control your emotions to win. Emotions have a profound effect on health and illness. Mind-body medicine studies show that thoughts and emotions influence health.

SUN TZU said:

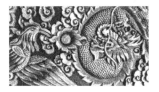

Generally, the principles of warfare are: The general receives his commands from the ruler, assembles the troops, mobilizes the army, and sets up camp.

There is nothing more difficult than armed struggle.

In armed struggle, the difficulty is turning the circuitous into the direct, and turning adversity into advantage.

Therefore, if you make the enemy's route circuitous and bait him with advantages, though you start out behind him, you will arrive before him. This is to know the calculations of the circuitous and of the direct.

Therefore, armed struggle has advantages, and armed struggle has risks. If the entire army mobilizes for an advantage, you will not arrive on time.

DR. CHAN says:

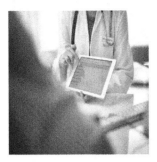

In health, there is nothing more difficult than fighting a serious disease. Do not look for conflict, look for opportunities. Look for different detours and paths (e.g., integrative medicine) to make sure your advantage is certain over disease, especially if confrontation is eminent. Don't move until you figure out the advantageous way to move. Some people see moving slowly as a form of weakness, but having control and good positioning is how to master energy, as well as power, emotions, and adaptability.

SUN TZU said:

If a reduced army mobilizes for an advantage, your stores and equipment will be lost.

For this reason, by rolling up your armor, rushing forward without stopping day or night, covering twice the usual distance for an advantage a hundred kilometers away, the general will be captured. The strong will arrive first, the weak will lag behind, and as a rule, only one-tenth will arrive.

If one struggles for an advantage fifty kilometers away, the general of the front forces will be thwarted, and as a rule only one half will arrive. If one struggles for an advantage thirty kilometers away, then two-thirds of the army will arrive.

For this reason, if an army is without its equipment it will lose; if an army is without its provisions it will lose; if the army is without its stores will lose.

DR. CHAN says:

If your health is reduced and you confront disease, you will lose something. Depending on how healthy you are and how prepared you are, will dictate how well you do in a battle against disease.

If you have not seen your healthcare providers, have not had regular screenings and testing, and have not maintained a healthy lifestyle, you will have a significant setback in your health if you have to battle disease.

SUN TZU said:

Therefore, one who does not know the intentions of the rulers of the neighboring states cannot secure alliances.

One who does not know the mountains and forests, gorges and defiles, swamps and wetlands cannot advance the army. One who does not use local guides cannot take advantage of the ground.

Therefore, the army is established on deception, mobilized by advantage, and changed through dividing up and consolidating the troops.

Therefore, it advances like the wind; it marches like the forest; it invades and plunders like fire; it stands like the mountain; it is formless like the dark; it strikes like thunder.

When you plunder the countryside, divide the wealth among your troops; when you expand your territory, divide up and hold places of advantage.

Calculate the situation, and then move. Those who know the principles of the circuitous and direct will be victorious. This is armed struggle.

DR. CHAN says:

One who does not have the knowledge about how disease operates, cannot collaborate with their healthcare providers to gain the advantage over disease. One who does not use their guides – physicians, nutritionists, fitness trainers, acupuncturists, massage therapists, and others – cannot have advantage over disease.

When you are knowledgeable about disease, mobilize your healthcare providers, and expand your areas of healthcare, you will have the advantage over disease.

In health, Sun Tzu's lesson is: do not hurry into battle. Look for advantageous alliances and good positioning in your healthcare. You must align with yourself first. Make sure you are not sabotaging yourself. It all begins with self-love. Mind-body medicine and journaling can help you communicate with yourself.

SUN TZU said:

The Book of Military Administration says: It is because words cannot be clearly heard in battle, drums and gongs are used; it is because troops cannot see each other clearly in battle, flags and pennants are used.

Therefore, in night battles use torches and drums; in day battles use flags and pennants. Drums, gongs, flags, and pennants are used to unite men's eyes and ears.

When the men are united, the brave cannot advance alone, the cowardly cannot retreat alone. These are the principles for employing a large number of troops.
Therefore, in night battles, use many torches and drums, and in day battles, use many flags and pennants in order to influence men's eyes and ears.

The energy of the army can be dampened, and the general's mind can be dampened. Therefore, in the morning, energy is high, but during the day energy begins to flag; and in the evening, energy is exhausted.

Therefore, those skilled in the use of force avoid [the enemy's] high energy, and strike when energy is exhausted. This is the way to manage energy.

DR. CHAN says:

When doing battle with disease, unite with your healthcare providers and use many forms of communication to stay connected with them - and with yourself. Be sure you and your providers communicate and understand each other and agree on the strategies to be used. Keep in communication with yourself by practicing mind/body medicine and journaling.

Manage your emotions and your energy level. Disease will look to strike when your energy is exhausted.

Mind-Body Medicine

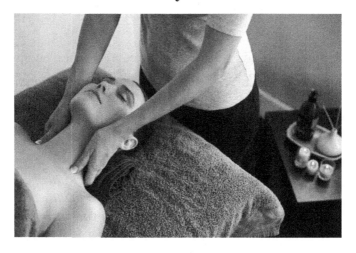

"The natural healing force within each one of us is the greatest force in getting well."

~Hippocrates

Mind-body medicine is based on the fact that how we think and feel affects our bodies. And our bodies, or what happens physically, can affect our thoughts and feelings. Mind-body medicine focuses on the interaction between the body, the mind, and behavior, and their effect on health and disease. It also focuses on the many factors that can affect health and wellbeing, including emotional, mental, social, spiritual, experiential, and behavioral factors. Mind-body techniques are designed to reduce stress, which can compromise immune function.

Ancient healing practices, such as Traditional Chinese Medicine and Ayurvedic medicine, emphasize the interaction between mind and body. Western medical views have emphasized the opposite – that the mind and body are separate. But those views are changing. There are many new studies that support mind-body medicine and, therefore, many new programs that are being established in top medical institutions nationally and internationally.

The History of Mind-Body Medicine

- *1964 - Psychiatrist George Solomon noted that patients with rheumatoid arthritis got worse when they were depressed. He studied the impact of emotions on inflammation and the immune system in general. The new field was called psychoneuroimmunology ("psycho" for psychology; "neuro" for neurology, or nervous system; and "immunology" for immunity).*

- *The 1960s and early 1970s - Herbert Benson, a cardiologist and founder of Harvard's Mind/Body Medicinal Institute, coined the term "relaxation response," after studying how meditation affects blood pressure. He found the relaxation response is basically the opposite reaction to the "fight or flight" response, and that using the response is beneficial because it counteracts the physiological effects of stress and the fight or flight response.*

- *1975 - Psychologist Robert Ader proved that mental and emotional cues could affect the immune system.*

- *1989 - David Spiegel, M.D. at Stanford University School of Medicine, demonstrated the power of the mind to heal. Of 86 women with late stage breast cancer, half received standard medical care while the other half received the standard care plus weekly support sessions. In these latter sessions, the women were able to share their experiences. Dr. Spiegel discovered that the women who participated in the social support group lived twice as long as the women who did not.*

- *Many clinical studies show that the patients who feel helplessness and hopelessness are associated with a lesser chance of survival.*

Mind-body Techniques

The key to mind-body techniques is to develop a state of "focused concentration," that triggers a relaxation response. According to Dr. Benson, one of the most valuable things we can do in life is to learn how to deeply relax. Make an effort every day to quiet your mind in order to create inner peace and better health. Some of the most commonly used techniques include:

- **Biofeedback** - *Through biofeedback, people can be trained to control certain bodily processes that normally occur involuntarily, such as heart rate or blood pressure. Biofeedback is effective for a number of conditions, including: headaches, migraines, chronic pain, anxiety, ADD/ADHD and others.*
- **Cognitive behavioral therapy** - *This technique is used to help people recognize and change negative thoughts.*
- **Meditation** – *A practice to help you quiet your mind and relax. It aids in focusing and becoming more aware.*
- **Visualization and Guided Imagery** – *A technique that uses images to help create focused relaxation.*
- **Progressive muscle relaxation** – *Tightening and relaxing muscles in progression to achieve deep relaxation.*
- **Acupuncture** – *A key component of ancient Chinese medicine, whereby thin needles are inserted in the top of the skin along meridians of the body. It is commonly used for pain relief, nausea, and other conditions.*
- **Energy healing** – *Tapping into the body's frequencies to promote healing, such as Reiki and Emotional Freedom Technique (EFT), whereby you tap along acupressure points to relieve stress.*

- **Massage** - *Massage is used for relaxation and well-being, and is also beneficial in treating injuries, other musculoskeletal issues, and many painful conditions.*
- **Breathing techniques** – *Deep breathing is an excellent way to relieve stress.*
- **Hypnosis or hypnotherapy** - *Using guided relaxation, hypnosis relaxes a person's body while their thoughts become focused. Hypnosis is used to treat people with addictions, pain, anxiety disorders, and phobias.*
- **Prayer and Spiritual Beliefs** - *Research suggests that qualities like faith, hope, and forgiveness, and using prayer and social support, have a significant effect on health and healing.*
- **Body movement** – *Yoga, Tai Chi, and exercise off all types, help physical conditioning, prevent disease, and improve a number of health problems, including: high blood pressure, cardiovascular disease, diabetes and arthritis. Physical movement is also considered vital for mental health. Research on anxiety and depression shows that body movement and exercise have psychological benefits, sometimes as great as medication, and the effects can be long lasting.*
- **Therapies for Art, Music, Dance, Laughter** – *Creative therapies can reduce stress and anxiety and bring a positive change in mood.*

How it works

When you are physically or emotionally stressed, your body releases stress hormones that can affect your entire body. For example, stress related to hostility and anxiety, can compromise the heart and immune system. Depression may also affect the immune system and affect the body's capacity to heal.

The goal of mind-body techniques is to get the body and mind to relax, which will reduce the levels of stress hormones in the body, and keep your immune system strong.

Mind-body techniques are helpful because, besides encouraging relaxation, they can help improve coping skills, reduce tension and pain, and therefore, lessen the need for medication.

Mind-body techniques may help treat many different diseases and disorders, including:
- *Cancer*
- *High blood pressure*
- *Asthma*
- *Coronary heart disease*
- *Obesity*
- *Pain and nausea related to chemotherapy*
- *Insomnia*
- *Diabetes*
- *Stomach and intestinal problems (including indigestion, irritable bowel syndrome, constipation, diarrhea, ulcerative colitis, heartburn, and Crohn's disease)*
- *Fibromyalgia*
- *Chronic fatigue syndrome*
- *Menopausal symptoms such as hot flashes, depression, and irritability*
- *Mental health issues, such as anxiety and depression*

SUN TZU said:

Disciplined, wait for disorder; calm, wait for clamor. This is the way to manage the mind.

Near, wait for the distant; rested, wait for the fatigued; full, wait for the hungry. This is the way to manage strength.

Do not do battle with well-ordered flags; do not do battle with well-regulated formations. This is the way to manage adaptation.

Therefore, the principles of warfare are: Do not attack an enemy that has the high ground; do not attack an enemy that has his back to a hill; do not pursue feigned retreats; do not attack elite troops; do not swallow the enemy's bait.

Do not thwart an enemy retreating home. If you surround the enemy, leave an outlet; do not press an enemy that is cornered. These are the principles of warfare.

DR. CHAN says:

We win against disease by staying disciplined and calm – having self-control and managing our mind.

Only do battle with disease when you are rested and well nourished, so you are strong.

Become adaptable when battling disease, so you can seize opportunities. Do not press disease - for example the overuse of antibiotics can lead to antibiotic resistance. It is not just your strength that matters, but your ability to see the opportunities for success.

2. Adaptability in Health

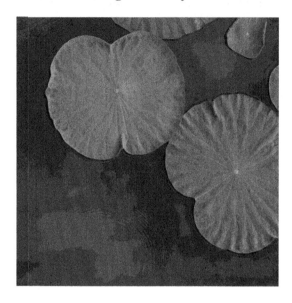

Sun Tzu teaches that we need to stay focused and consistent, but constantly evaluate and change our plans in order to be successful. It is the same with health. We need to be adaptable, achieving small results over time to be healthy and to stay on top of disease. To achieve optimal health - be proactive, instead of reactive in your healthcare.

Invest in the health services you need now to thwart disease. Your character will determine your adaptability.

SUN TZU said:

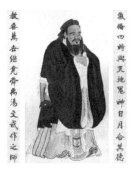

Generally, the principles of warfare are: The general receives his commands from the ruler, assembles the armies, and mobilizes the masses.

Do not camp on difficult ground. Unite with your allies on intersecting ground. Do not stay on open ground. Be prepared on surrounded ground. Do battle on deadly ground.

There are routes not to be taken; there are armies not to be attacked; there are walled cities not to be besieged; there are grounds not to be penetrated; there are commands not to be obeyed.

Therefore, the general who knows the advantages of the nine changes knows how to use the troops.

If the general does not know the advantages of the nine changes, even if he knows the lay of the land, he will not be able to take advantage of the ground.

DR. CHAN says:

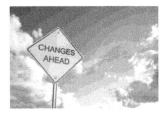

You and your healthcare providers can use adaptability to your advantage - to seize opportunities over disease. When Sun Tzu writes about the general who knows about the nine changes, he means a leader who can create many options for himself and his army. When you and your healthcare providers are adaptable, you have the freedom to choose various options, either conventional or integrative, that will benefit you.

The leader who does not know the nine (many) changes, even though he knows other things (the lay of the land), will not be able to gain advantage in the battle. When you and your healthcare providers are not open to options and change, you are handicapped and your health outcomes will not be as advantageous as they could be.

SUN TZU said:

He who commands an army but does not know the principles of the nine changes, even if he is familiar with the five advantages, will not be able to best use his troops.

Therefore, the intelligent general contemplates both the advantages and disadvantages.

Contemplating the advantages, he fulfills his calculations; contemplating the disadvantages, he removes his difficulties.

Therefore, subjugate the neighboring rulers with potential disadvantages, labor the neighboring rulers with constant matters, and have the neighboring rulers rush after advantages.

So the principles of warfare are: Do not depend on the enemy not coming, but depend on our readiness against him. Do not depend on the enemy not attacking, but depend on our position that cannot be attacked.

DR. CHAN says:

The intelligent healthcare provider and patient are skilled in thinking about not only the options of healthcare, but both the advantages and disadvantages of moving forward with any healthcare situation. Creativity should be an important part of the approach to your healthcare. Adjust the methods to address your specific situation. Be proactive in your healthcare to have an advantage, rather than reactive and then have to do serious battle when you may not be ready.

Do not assume that you will not become ill, but be prepared for illness at any time – prepare for the worst. Aim for optimal health, so there are areas where you cannot be attacked.

SUN TZU said:

Therefore, there are five dangerous traits of a general:

He who is reckless can be killed.
He who is cowardly can be captured.
He who is quick tempered can be insulted.
He who is moral can be shamed.
He who is fond of the people can be worried.

These five traits are faults in a general, and are disastrous in warfare. The army's destruction, and the death of the general, are due to these five dangerous traits. They must be examined.

DR. CHAN says:

In the first chapter, Sun Tzu lists the five traits of a leader – smart, trustworthy, caring, brave, and disciplined. In keeping with yin and yang, this chapter looks at the opposite and addresses the extremes of these traits that become faults and therefore dangerous when doing battle. These dangerous traits are:

Smart becomes fearfulness and analyzing too much.
Trustworthy becomes too sensitive.
Caring becomes too attached.
Brave becomes fearless and too aggressive.
Disciplined becomes too strict and hot tempered.

Adaptability is basically a decision making skill. As our own healthcare leaders, we must keep an eye on our leadership skills and traits, because they set the course for our healthcare decisions and our life.

Wellness Warrior Actions: Week 7

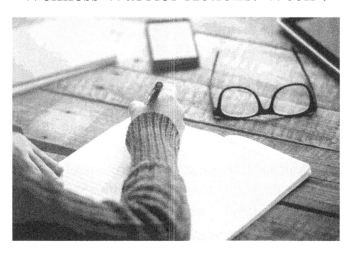

Vision Meditation

- Have your journal ready to record your thoughts after you meditate.
- Sit in a private, quiet, and comfortable place.
- Close your eyes and relax.
- Take a deep breath in and exhale three times to empty the air in your chest (this will start your deep breathing).
- Take a breath for each number and count backwards from 10 to 1, as you relax your body and center yourself. Notice where there is tension and let it go with your breath.
- Think about how your week went. How did you do on the past week's goal or goals?
- Is there anything you would have done differently?
- **For week 7** – Meditate on confrontation and adaptability in your healthcare. Are you being proactive and investing in your future health to avoid a serious health battle? Are you using your guides and healthcare providers? Who are they, and could you seek other guides to aid you? Are there additional options you could seek to have optimal health? What are those areas and options?
- What area or areas in Mind-Body Medicine could you pursue to relieve stress and improve your health? See yourself as an

adaptable leader of your health, possessing the traits needed to be successful:
Smart, but not fearful,
Trustworthy, but not too sensitive.
Caring, but not too attached.
Brave, but not fearless or too aggressive.
Disciplined, but not too strict and hot tempered.

- Refer back to your healthy vision. Begin to see what it would look like in the future if you were more adaptable in your healthcare, if you were proactive and looked at options that would give you optimal health. See yourself as an adaptable leader of your health – disciplined, brave, creative and caring. Envision yourself doing various types of mind-body medicine. What would that look like a few months from now, a year from now, 10 years from now? See yourself as very healthy. What does that look like? What does that feel like?

Journaling:
- Write "Week 7" in your journal and record what you accomplished this week in keeping your goal or goals. Write any observations you may have and what you may want to do differently in the future.

This week's goals:
- Write down the health areas and options you want to pursue in order to be adaptable and proactive, that will position you for any health confrontation, and that will continue to move you forward to optimal health. Is it to contact a healthcare provider or guide? Sign up for a program or plan? Practicing mind-body medicine? What traits do you need to work on to be an adaptable leader for your health? More self-caring or braver? Write them down. Which steps could you take to improve these traits? Since we are taking small steps to achieve optimal health, be sure to follow the 80/20 Rule -

what is the 20% you could do that would give you 80% of the results you want? Write your 20% action as a goal or goals. Make sure it's a SMART goal.

S – Specific: What exactly do you want to do? Clearly define your goal.
M – Measurable: How can you measure and track progress?
A – Attainable: Can you achieve it in the time frame?
R – Relevant: Is it relevant to your long-term goals?
T – Time bound: When will you take action?

"So the principles of warfare are: Do not depend on the enemy not coming, but depend on our readiness against him. Do not depend on the enemy not attacking, but depend on our position that cannot be attacked."

~ Sun Tzu

WEEK 8

COMPETITIVE ENVIRONMENTS IN HEALTHCARE

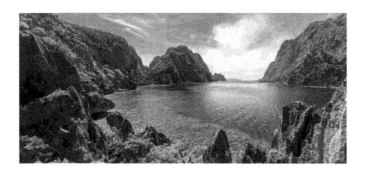

We live in a competitive universe. Life is about competition. Sun Tzu explains four different competitive environments and how to use them. For our purposes, these dimensions represent different areas of health and healthcare. One dimension is ideal for maintaining good health.

The four environments are:
1. **Level Ground** (Stable, Neutral, Predictable) – Ideal environment for maintaining good health, plateaus.
2. **Marshes** (Soft, Unpredictable) – Diseases
3. **Water** (Fluid, Unstable) – New trends in healthcare and drugs.
4. **Mountains** (Tilted, Uneven) – Doctors, healthcare system, insurance.

We'll look at each environment and determine how we can use each one for our health advantage.

SUN TZU said:

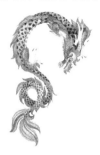

Generally, on positioning the army and observing the enemy:
To cross mountains, stay close to the valleys; observe on high ground and face the sunny side. If the enemy holds the high ground, do not ascend and do battle with him. This is positioning the army in the mountains.

After crossing a river, you must stay far away from it. If the enemy crosses a river, do not meet him in the water. When half of his forces has crossed, it will then be advantageous to strike.

If you want to do battle with the enemy, do not position your forces near the water facing the enemy; take high ground facing the sunny side, and do not position downstream. This is positioning the army near rivers.

After crossing swamps and wetlands, strive to quickly get through them, and do not linger. If you do battle in swamps and wetlands, you must position close to grass, with the trees to your back. This is positioning the army in swamps and wetlands.

On level ground, position on places that are easy to maneuver with your right backed by high ground, with the dangerous ground in front, and safe ground to the back. This is positioning the army on level ground.

These are the four positions advantageous to the army, which enabled the Yellow Emperor to conquer four rulers.

DR. CHAN says:

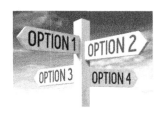

Mountains are uneven, complicated terrains, with many variations. They are: healthcare providers, the current healthcare system, and insurers. They can be hard to navigate and range from small organizations and practices to large bureaucracies.

Water is not stable. It represents current trends in medicine: current nutrition, exercise, medication, and testing recommendations. These are trends that are always changing.

Marshes and swamps represent disease. You want to move quickly through swamps, (disease), because you don't want it to develop into something chronic, because it takes a toll on your body, and can also be costly.

Level ground, or plateaus, is the ideal environment for good health. It is a stable environment to maintain good health and use the advantages of the other environments to position yourself. It includes: integrative medicine, functional medicine, and mind-body medicine. Level ground is easy to navigate so you can position yourself for success, staying healthy and avoiding disease.

SUN TZU said:

Generally, the army prefers high ground and dislikes low ground, values the sunny side and despises the shady side, nourishes its health and occupies places with resources, and avoids numerous sicknesses. These factors mean certain victory.

Where there are hills and embankments, you must position on the sunny side, with the hills and embankments to your right back.

These are advantages to the army.

Use the ground for assistance.

When the rainwater rises and descends down to where you want to cross, wait until it settles.

Where there is ground with impassable ravines, Heaven's Wells, Heaven's Prisons, Heaven's Nets, Heaven's Pits, and Heaven's Fissures, you must march quickly away from them. Do not approach them.

When we distance from them, draw the enemy to approach them. When we move to face the enemy, he will have them at his back.

When the army is flanked by high ground, wetlands, tall reeds and grass, mountain forests, or areas with thick undergrowth, you must search carefully and thoroughly, because these are places where men lie in ambush or where spies hide.

If the enemy is close and remains quiet, he occupies a natural stronghold.

If the enemy is far away and challenges you to do battle, he wants you to advance, because he occupies level ground that is to his advantage.

DR. CHAN says:

Certain victory in health is brought about by being proactive - positioning and nourishing yourself, and using your resources to avoid illness.

You must constantly be aware of the environment - paying attention to the details and making sure you are on level ground, adjusting to be sure you have the advantage over illness. You must search thoroughly and carefully, to be sure that illness is not hiding and waiting in ambush and that you are not engaging in self-sabotage. Pay attention so you don't revert back to old habits or old-brain thinking.

When disease is close and quiet it can occupy a stronghold. Don't let illness maintain level ground and have the advantage.

SUN TZU said:

If trees move, he is advancing; if there are obstacles placed in the undergrowth, he wants to make us suspicious.

If the birds take flight, he is lying in ambush; if the animals are in fear, he is preparing to attack.

If dust is high in straight columns, his chariots are advancing; if dust is low and wide, his infantry is advancing. If the dust is scattered, he is gathering wood; if the dust is sparse, coming and going, he is encamping.

If he speaks humbly, but increases warfare readiness, he will advance.

If he speaks belligerently and advances aggressively, he will retreat.

If he speaks apologetically, he needs a rest.

If his light chariots move first and take position on the flanks, he is setting up for battle. If he seeks peace without a treaty, he is calculating.

If he sets up his troops rapidly, he is expecting reinforcements.

If half of his troops advances and half of his troops retreats, he is trying to lure you.

If the troops lean on their weapons, they are hungry. If the troops who draw water drink first, they are thirsty.

If he sees advantage but does not take it, he is tired.

If birds gather, he is not there.

If his troops cry at night, they are afraid.

If the army is unsettled, the general is weak.

If the enemy's flags and pennants move about, he is in chaos.

If the officers are irritable, they are exhausted.

If his horses are fed grain and his men meat, no longer hangs up cooking pots, and does not return to camp, he is desperate.

If troops constantly gather in small groups and whisper together, he has lost his men.

If he gives out rewards frequently, he is running out of resources.

If he gives out punishments frequently, he is dire straits.

If he is brutal at first, and then fears the masses, he is the extreme of ineptitude.

If he comes with offerings, he wants to rest.

If his troops confront you with anger, but do not do battle or leave their position, he must be investigated.

DR. CHAN says:

You must know the nature and signs of disease. Pay attention to the details and nuances. The different environments can be advantageous for you.

Mountains, *or conventional medicine, possess power and importance, especially for life-threatening conditions.*

Water, *or new trends, can offer alternatives especially for chronic conditions.*

Marshes, *or disease, can have plateaus that can be advantageous.*

When you are on ***level ground*** *be proactive and position yourself.*
Be suspicious and continually look for signs of disease so you don't have to do serious battle.

Watch for signs or symptoms of illness:
- *low energy*
- *changes in your appetite*
- *too thirsty*
- *urinate too frequently*
- *pain*
- *shortness of breath*
- *heart palpitations*
- *skin changes or rashes*
- *bowel changes*
- *constant cough*
- *changes in vision*
- *signs of an infection or flu-like symptoms*

- *insomnia*
- *confusion*

SUN TZU said:

In warfare, numbers may not necessarily be an advantage; do not advance aggressively.

It is enough to consolidate your strength, calculate the enemy, and get support from your men.

One who lacks strategic planning and underestimates the enemy will be captured.

If one punishes the troops before their loyalty is formed, they will be disobedient. If they are disobedient, they will be difficult to use. If one does not punish the troops after their loyalty is formed, they cannot be used.

Therefore, if he commands them by benevolence, and unifies them by discipline, this is called certain victory.

If commands are consistently enforced when training men, they will be obedient; if commands are not consistently enforced when training men, they will be disobedient.

If commands are consistently executed, they are in accord with the general.

DR. CHAN says:

In health, your numbers may not necessarily be an advantage. Do not assume that because the numbers on your blood work, blood pressure, etc. are normal, that you can move forward aggressively, or let down your guard. While these are good signs, you still have to be on the alert. Do not underestimate the enemy and abandon strategic planning for your health.

Be sure and watch for self-sabotage. Self-sabotage may occur when you are on level ground and you think you do not have to position yourself for future health. Love yourself enough to live a healthy lifestyle, stay in good communication with your healthcare providers, monitor for disease and continue to take small steps toward optimal health.

Self-sabotage and the strategy to change it

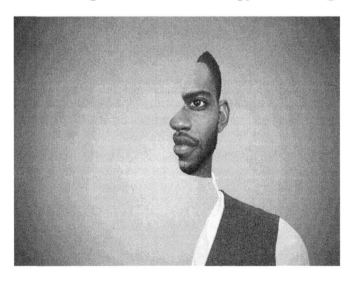

Self-sabotage impacts most people's lives in some way. It encompasses reoccurring negative thoughts, feelings, attitudes, and behaviors. It is a repetitive pattern of behavior that results in unintended and harmful consequences.

Those who engage in a repetitive cycle of failed attempts to fulfill a need—may be vulnerable to mental health difficulties, such as depression and anxiety. They share in the frustration of having a need unfulfilled, and diminished self-efficacy in future attempts to change. Self-sabotage may reflect a self-perpetuating negative spiral in which the more one attempts to fulfill an unmet need, the greater the resulting sense of frustration.

Origins of Self-sabotage

Self-defeating behaviors originate from negative beliefs that you are not adequate in some way. They stem from fear.

Changing Self-sabotage

To change a self-defeating behavior you must first recognize it and state what the behavior is. Then you can have insight into the thoughts, feelings and beliefs that lead to the behavior. Assess the harmful consequences and understand their origins to bolster your motivation and change to healthy alternative behaviors.

- *Identify self-sabotage behaviors and patterns without criticism, but with a feeling of self-love and self-help.*
- *Recognize the self-defeating consequences. How do these behaviors negatively impact your life? What is the price you pay? See the behavior as an unsuccessful attempt to satisfy a need or pattern that relieved anxiety.*
- *Understand the origin of the self-sabotage. Understanding the negative pattern will help you see the underlying need, the core belief and the life circumstance which led to the behavior. This should also help in the process of changing to a healthier behavior.*
- *Identify the unfulfilled need or negative belief that prompted the behavior, so you can change to a healthier behavior.*
- *Develop an alternative belief and behavior pattern. The goal is to increase recognition of the situations and factors that contribute to the self-sabotage pattern. Monitor self-*

thought and see how it contributes to behavior. Stop negative thoughts and replace with positive thoughts, beliefs and behaviors.

- *Develop alternative healthy behaviors and attempt to test them, taking small steps as you experiment with alternatives.*
- *Document situations. Document your thoughts, feelings, behaviors, and situations in which the self-sabotaging patterns are activated. Make deliberate choices to reflect self-encouraging beliefs about yourself.*
- *Change your response. Now that you recognize how a core belief created a behavior, create some time before you respond to a situation. Rather than acting out a feeling, act out your deliberate choice. Develop the ability to tolerate the new choice.*
- *Change the core belief. Delete the self-sabotaging core beliefs and replace them with a self-enhancing belief. As you learn to tolerate your new choices and use alternative responses, you will probably come to realize that the original belief has lost its value*
- *Preventing self-defeating behaviors in the future - is a lifelong process. Evaluating your life and patterns of behavior is a lifelong process. Meditating and journaling are lifelong sources of support you can use to maintain healthy patterns of behavior. They can help in identifying and changing any self-defeating behaviors.*

Wellness Warrior Actions: Week 8

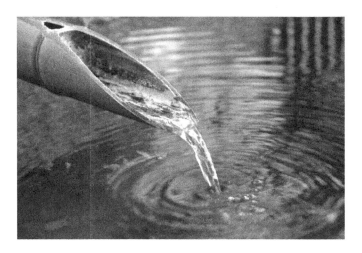

Vision Meditation
- Have your journal ready to record your thoughts after you meditate.
- Sit in a private, quiet, and comfortable place.
- Close your eyes and relax.
- Take a deep breath in and exhale three times to empty the air in your chest (this will start your deep breathing).
- Take a breath for each number and count backwards from 10 to 1, as you relax your body and center yourself. Notice where there is tension and let it go with your breath.
- Think about how your week went. How did you do on the past week's goal or goals?
- Is there anything you would have done differently?
- **For week 8** – Meditate on which environment/environments you are in right now. Are you in the marshes with disease? In water and going through changes? In the mountains? On level ground and positioning yourself for a healthy future by being proactive? Are you in a few environments? Are you self-sabotaging yourself in any areas of your health? What are they?
- Refer back to your healthy vision. Begin to see what it would look like in the future if you changed some of the

environments you are in, worked on any areas of self-sabotage and supported your optimal health. What would that look like a few months from now, a year from now, 10 years from now? See yourself as very healthy. What does that look like? What does that feel like?

Journaling

- Write "Week 8" in your journal and record what you accomplished this week in keeping your goal or goals. Write any observations you may have and what you may want to do differently in the future.

This week's goals

- Write down what environment/environments you are in. What do you need to do to get on a plateau? If you are on a plateau, are you doing what you need to do to position yourself for your future healthy self? Are you paying attention and on the alert for any enemies – disease or yourself? Are you self-sabotaging yourself in any way by not doing what you could do for optimal health?
- Go through the self-sabotaging article above and document any self-sabotaging behaviors you have towards your health – anything you are doing or not doing that doesn't lead to your optimal health. In a spirit of exploration and self-love, follow the strategy for changing self-sabotage and document your findings, as you identify and begin to change your behavior this week.

"Love yourself enough to live a healthy lifestyle."
~ Dr. Kevin Chan

WEEK 9

EVALUATING OPPORTUNITIES IN

HEALTH

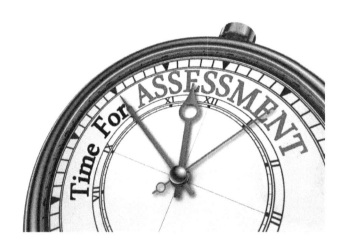

Sun Tzu explained six opportunities you can use to evaluate your position in moving forward or defending yourself. We will look at these dimensions and how you can use them when moving forward toward optimal health while defending yourself against disease.

The six dimensions are complementary opposites which are an extension of the five elements. The three dimensions: areas, obstacles, and dangers - and their complementary opposites - represent every strategic opportunity or position. Some positions are meant for moving forward and some are meant for defense.

The six dimensions of positioning are:

Areas/Distance:
1. Spread out – Far
2. Constricted – Close, unity, focused

Obstruction/Obstacles:
3. Wide-open/Accessible – Easy to get to
4. Barricaded – Hard to get to

Dangers/Holding power:

5. Entangling – Difficult to leave
6. Supportive – Don't want to leave

SUN TZU said:

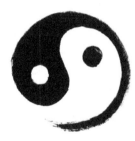

The grounds are accessible, entrapping, stalemated, narrow, steep, and expansive. If you can go through but the enemy cannot, it is called accessible.

For accessible ground, first take the high and the sunny side, and convenient supply routes. You then do battle with the advantage.

If you can go through but difficult to go back, it is called entrapping. For entrapping ground, if the enemy is unprepared, advance and defeat him.

If the enemy is prepared, and you advance and are not victorious, it will be difficult to go back; this is disadvantageous.

If it is not advantageous to advance or for the enemy to advance, it is called stalemated. For stalemated ground, though the enemy offers you advantage, do not advance. Withdraw.

If you strike them when half has advanced, this is advantageous.

DR. CHAN says:

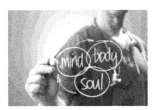

The six dimensions are metaphysical positions to help you examine what is advantageous for your health. The dimensions correlate with weaknesses. When you are in certain situations, it exposes your weakness. You need to know your character, when evaluating health opportunities, so you can choose which position is right for you. Every position has advantages and disadvantages for individuals.

SUN TZU said:

For narrow ground, we must occupy it first; be prepared and wait for the enemy. If the enemy occupies it first, and is prepared, do not follow him. If he is not prepared, follow him.

For steep ground, if you occupy it first, occupy the high on the sunny side and wait for the enemy. If the enemy occupies it first, withdraw; do not follow him.

For expansive ground, if the forces are equal, it will be difficult to do battle. Doing battle will not be advantageous. These are the six Ways of ground. They are the general's responsibility, and must be examined.

DR. CHAN says:

These are the six health positions. Keep in mind that certain positions are advantageous for certain people and hurt others. In exploring and finding the right position for you, you will learn more about yourself and be able to choose wisely when assessing future strategic positions.

The six positions help you to know where you are at any given time in relation to disease. Are you moving forward, waiting, attacking, or defending?

Areas/Distance:

1. ***Spread out – Far:*** *In this position where many things are spread out or far away, you need to handle tasks without overextending yourself or spreading yourself too thin. If you do overextend yourself, you will be surprised by disease.*

2. ***Constricted – Close, unity, focused:*** *The constricted position is one that requires focus and unity. If you cannot stay focused, in this position you will usually have self-doubts, which will lead to self-destruction or self-sabotage.*

Obstruction/Obstacles:

3. ***Wide-open/Accessible – Easy to get to:*** *When you are in a wide-open position, things are easily accessible and it's easy to maneuver. But, you can become clumsy and then potentially outmaneuvered by disease. Therefore, you must take care not to be clumsy when things are easy.*

4. ***Barricaded – Hard to get to:*** *If you are barricaded, it is a good position because it will be hard for disease to get to you, and easy to defend. Therefore, you must be organized. If you are disorganized, then disease can besiege you.*

Dangers/Holding power:

5. **Entangling – Difficult to leave:** *When you are in an entangled position, it is difficult to leave, therefore you must be disciplined and do what needs to be done. If you are not disciplined, you could be hurt.*
6. **Supportive – Don't want to leave:** *A supportive position can be a very good position unless you are not knowledgeable and don't know what you are doing. You need to be knowledgeable, in order to take a supportive position against disease.*

SUN TZU said:

In warfare, there are six situations: flight, insubordination, deterioration, collapse, chaos, and setback. These situations are not caused by Heaven or Ground, but by the general.

If the forces are equal, and one attacks ten, this is called flight. If the troops are strong but the officers weak, this is called insubordination. If the officers are strong but the troops weak, this is called deterioration.

If the officers are angry and insubordinate, doing battle with the enemy under anger and insubordination, and the general does not know their abilities, this is called collapse.

If the general is weak and not disciplined, his instructions not clear, the officers and troops lack discipline and their formation in disarray, this is called chaos.

If the general cannot calculate his enemy, and uses a small number against a large number, his weak attacking the strong, and has no selected vanguard, this is called setback. These are the six Ways of defeat. They are the general's responsibility, and must be examined.

DR. CHAN says:

There are six weaknesses that correlate with the six dimensions. These weaknesses are due to bad decisions made by you or your healthcare providers. Poor decisions place you in a bad position, at the wrong time. Stay alert to be sure you are not putting yourself in a bad position.

1. ***Spread out/Far*** *– exposes overextension leading to flight.*
2. ***Constricted*** *- exposes self-destruction leading to collapse.*
3. ***Wide-open/Accessible*** *– exposes clumsiness leading to setback.*
4. ***Barricaded*** *– exposes disorganization leading to chaos.*
5. ***Entangling*** *- exposes lack of discipline leading to insubordination.*
6. ***Supportive*** *– exposes lack of training leading to deterioration.*

SUN TZU said:

Those who do battle and know these are certain for victory. Those who do battle and do not know these are certain for defeat.

Therefore, if the Way of warfare indicates certain victory, though the ruler does not want to do battle, the general may do battle. If the Way of warfare indicates defeat, though the ruler wants to do battle, the general may not do battle.

Therefore, the general who does not advance to seek glory, or does not withdraw to avoid punishment, but cares for only the people's security and promotes the people's interests, is the nation's treasure.

He looks upon his troops as children, and they will advance to the deepest valleys. He looks upon his troops as his own children, and they will die with him.

If the general is kind to the troops, but cannot use them, or if the general loves the troops, but cannot command them, or if the general does not discipline the troops, but cannot establish order, the troops are like spoiled children and are useless.

DR. CHAN says:

When choosing a healthcare provider, you want one who is not only disciplined and caring, but someone who also knows when to do battle.

If the healthcare provider is knowledgeable, disciplined, and has your interests at heart, and if they treat you as a family member – they are a treasure.

If the healthcare provider is lacking in any of these areas, then you will not know victory over disease.

SUN TZU said:

If I know the troops can attack, but do not know the enemy cannot attack, my victory is half.

If I know the enemy can be attacked, but do not know the troops cannot attack, my victory is half.

If I know the enemy can be attacked, and know the troops can attack, but do not know the ground in battle, my victory is half.

Therefore, one who knows how to advance the army is limitless when taking action.
Therefore I say, if you know the enemy and know yourself, the victory is not at risk. If you know the Heaven and you know the Ground, the victory is complete.

DR. CHAN says:

If you know yourself and the enemy (disease), then optimal health can be yours. If you know the six positions and how to use them, your victory will be complete.

Wellness Warrior Actions: Week 9

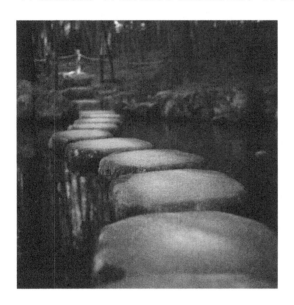

Vision Meditation

- Have your journal ready to record your thoughts after you meditate.
- Sit in a private, quiet, and comfortable place.
- Close your eyes and relax.
- Take a deep breath in and exhale three times to empty the air in your chest (this will start your deep breathing).
- Take a breath for each number and count backwards from 10 to 1, as you relax your body and center yourself. Notice where there is tension and let it go with your breath.
- Think about how your week went. How did you do on the past week's goal or goals?

- Is there anything you would have done differently?
- **For week 9**– Meditate on your positioning of healthcare in the six dimensions. Go through each dimension to see how they pertain to you.

The six dimensions of positioning:

Areas/Distance:
1. Spread out – Far
2. Constricted – Close, unity, focused

Obstruction/Obstacles:
3. Wide-open/Accessible – Easy to get to
4. Barricaded – Hard to get to

Dangers/Holding power:
5. Entangling – Difficult to leave
6. Supportive – Don't want to leave

- Refer back to your healthy vision. Begin to see what it would look like in the future if you evaluated what dimensions you are in now and began to make healthy decisions based on those positions. What would that look like a few months from now, a year from now, 10 years from now? See yourself as very healthy due to this new knowledge. What does that look like? What does that feel like?

Journaling
- Write "Week 9" in your journal and record what you accomplished this week in keeping your goal or goals. Write any observations you may have and what you may want to do differently in the future.

This week's goals

- Write down each dimension and a goal that will either move you forward with your health or help defend you against disease. For example: Accessible and easy to get to – maybe you need to change doctors so they are easier to get to (whether that means closer proximity to you or they have office hours that are more convenient for you), or choose one who can communicate easier with you. Barricaded and hard to get to – maybe you need to stop buying certain unhealthy foods and mentally barricade yourself from that grocery aisle. List what those foods are and what you could buy instead that would be healthy and appetizing. Another would be to mentally barricade the elevator and take the stairs to your office instead. Go through each dimension and make it work for you with a positive goal.

Be sure and write your goals as SMART goals.

S – Specific: What exactly do you want to do? Clearly define your goal.

M – Measurable: How can you measure and track progress?

A – Attainable: Can you achieve it in the time frame?

R – Relevant: Is it relevant to your long-term goals?

T – Time bound: When will you take action? Time sensitive goals are more likely to be achieved than a loose thought of action without an end time attached to it.

"Therefore, the general - who does not advance to seek glory, or does not withdraw to avoid punishment, but cares for only the people's security and promotes the people's interests, is the nation's treasure."

~ Sun Tzu

WEEK 10

STAGES OF HEALTH SITUATIONS

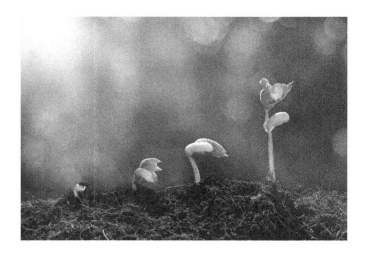

Sun Tzu explains nine situations, or stages of change in relation to conflict and the correct reaction to control each situation. These can apply to health and stages of change that can lead to optimal health. We'll review the stages of Sun Tzu, of Chinese medicine, as well as the stages of behavioral change in current medicine.

Sun Tzu teaches that each situation has a strategy. If you understand the stages of a situation, and which stage you are in, you can know what strategies to use. Using Sun Tzu's strategies as a model, you have a road map of how to improve your health.

In Chinese medicine, health is the balance of yin and yang. These are the two forces in all of nature, the complementary opposites: front and back, left and right, top and bottom, day and night. They are constant and ever changing. Chinese medicine strives to find the imbalances and correct them.

Traditional Chinese Medicine is comparable to conventional western medicine – it is a good start to routinely engage. **Classical Chinese Medicine,** on the other hand, is comparable to Integrative Medicine; it is broader in its scope and used to win.

Traditional Chinese Medicine is a modern modification of ancient Chinese medicine. It is a simpler form that was created in the 1940's. It is an adaptation of the pure form of Chinese Medicine, called Classical Chinese Medicine, which was formed 2000+ years ago.

Classical Chinese medicine is a specialty of Chinese medicine and practitioners require additional training in order to practice. You could say that Traditional Chinese Medicine practitioners are comparable to General Practitioners and Classical Chinese Medicine practitioners are comparable to specialists.

The diagnostic and therapeutic basics of Classical Chinese Medicine consist of six stages or levels: 3 yin, and 3 yang stages. The stages come in sequence, though you may not experience all stages for every situation. They chronicle the effects of a pathogen invasion from the exterior of the body to the interior. In summary the stages are:

Three Yang stages or levels:
- Tai Yang – posterior of the body (neck and head)
- Yang Ming - anterior of the body (face, abdomen)
- Shao Yang – lateral areas of the body (abdomen)

Three Yin Stages or levels:
- Tai Yin – the lung and spleen
- Shao Yin – the heart and kidney
- Jue Yin – the liver area

Each stage has its own treatment, which may include heat, cold, and flushing or detoxifying.

SUN TZU said:

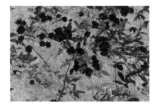

The principles of warfare are: There are dispersive ground, marginal ground, contentious ground, open ground, intersecting ground, critical ground, difficult ground, surrounded ground, and deadly ground.

Where the rulers do battle in their own ground, this is called dispersive ground. Where one enters the other's ground but not deep, this is called marginal ground. Where it is advantageous if you occupy it and it is advantageous if the enemy occupies it, this is called contentious ground. Where one can come and go, this is called open ground.

Where ground is surrounded by others, and the first one to reach it will gain the support of the masses, this is called intersecting ground. Where one enters deep into enemy ground, with many walled cities and towns to his back, this is called critical ground. Where there are mountains and forests, defiles and ravines, swamps and wetlands, and places difficult to pass, this is called difficult ground.

Where the entrance is narrow, the exit circuitous, allowing the enemy to attack his few to our many, this is called surrounded ground. Where if one who does battle with full force survives, and one who does not do battle with full force perishes, this is called deadly ground. Therefore,

1. On dispersive ground, do not do battle.
2. On marginal ground, do not stop.
3. On contentious ground, do not attack.
4. On open ground, do not become separated.

5. On intersecting ground, form alliances.
6. On critical ground, plunder.
7. On difficult ground, press on.
8. On surrounded ground, be prepared.
9. On deadly ground, do battle.

DR. CHAN says:

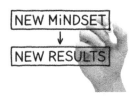

*Sun Tzu teaches there are **nine** stages or situations (grounds) that occur in sequence: early stages, middle stages, and late stages:*

Early Stage

1. <u>Dispersive ground:</u> *Scattered conditions. You may be scattered or you may have several areas of health concerns, often triggered by unexpected health events, or several healthcare providers.*
2. <u>Easy ground:</u> *You can make progress without struggle.*
3. <u>Contested ground</u>: *This is where you must engage (ill health) in competition for power.*

Middle Stage

4. <u>Open ground</u>: *Unobstructed conditions.*
5. <u>Shared ground</u>: *You share your healthcare and optimal health with healthcare providers, family and friends.*
6. <u>Dangerous ground</u>: *Conditions are not supporting your health, or you are not supporting your health.*

Late Stage

7. <u>*Difficult ground*</u>: *Things are not easy. You are having struggles in your life and/or health.*
8. <u>*Limited ground*</u>: *This can be a transitional or vulnerable stage that may include self-doubt and negative self-talk.*
9. <u>*Deadly ground*</u>: *You are in the clutches of disease and it is do or die.*

SUN TZU said:

In ancient times, those skilled in warfare were able to prevent the unity of the enemy's front and back, the many and the few, the noble and the peasants, and the superiors and the subordinates.

Have the enemy be separated and unable to assemble; if the enemy is assembled, it should not be organized.

Move when advantageous, stop when not advantageous.

Ask: If the enemy is large in number and advances, what should be the response?

I say: Seize what he values, and he will do what you wish.

The essential factor in warfare is speed.

To take advantage of the enemy's lack of preparation, take unexpected routes to attack where the enemy is not prepared.

Generally, the Way of invading is when one has penetrated deep into enemy ground, the troops are united; the defender will not be able to prevail.

DR. CHAN says:

In health, become skilled at preventing disease. You don't want to fight disease, you want to disorganize disease. If you have to fight, do it quickly. Attack disease where it is not prepared. Invade deep into enemy ground, which means to deeply commit to promoting optimal health and preventing disease. Do not let it invade your ground.

SUN TZU said:

If you plunder the fertile fields, the army will have enough provisions.

If you take care of your health, avoid fatigue, you will be united, and will build strength.

When moving troops and calculating plans, be formless.

Throw your troops into situations where there is no escape, where they will die before escaping. When they are about to die, what can they not do? They will exert their full strength.

When the troops are in desperate situations, they fear nothing; having penetrated deep in enemy ground, they are united.

When there are no other alternatives, they will fight.

Therefore, though not disciplined, they are alert; though not asked, they are devoted; though without promises, they are faithful; and though not commanded, they are trustworthy.

Prohibit omens, and get rid of doubts, and they will die without any other thoughts.

The soldiers do not have wealth, but not because they dislike material goods; they do not live long, but not because they dislike longevity.

On the day the men are issued orders to do battle, the sitting soldiers' tears will soak their sleeves, and the lying soldiers' tears will roll down their cheeks.

However, if you throw them into a desperate situation, they will have the courage of Chuan Chu or Ts'ao Kuei.

Therefore, those skilled in warfare are like the shuaijan. The shuaijan is a serpent on Mount Chang. If you strike its head, its tail attacks; if you strike its tail, its head attacks; if you strike its middle, both the head and tail attack.

Ask: Can forces be made like the shuaijan? I say: They can. The men of Wu and Yueh hated each other, however, encountering severe winds when crossing a river on the same boat, they assisted each other like left and right hands.

Therefore, hobbling horses and burying chariot wheels are not enough.

The Way of organization is uniting their courage, making the best of the strong and the weak through the principles of Ground.

Therefore, one who is skilled in warfare leads them by the hand like they are one person; they cannot but follow.

DR. CHAN says:

"If you take care of your health, avoid fatigue, you will be united, and will build strength."

You will be united holistically - in that your old brain and your new brain will be as one. Take care of your health and avoid fatigue and you will be united, in that there won't be any self-sabotage. Your strengths and weaknesses will unite to support you.

Your old brain is trying to protect you from any big changes. Use the art of deception for this and make small changes. The only way to make long term change is to make small steady changes.

SUN TZU said:

It is important for a general to be calm and remote, upright and disciplined, and be able to mystify his men's eyes and ears, keeping them ignorant.

He changes his methods and plans, keeping them from knowing. He changes his campsites and takes circuitous routes, keeping them from anticipating.

The day the general leads his troops into battle, it is like climbing up high and throwing away the ladder.

He leads his troops deep into enemy ground, and releases the trigger. He burns his boats and destroys the cooking pots.

He commands his troops like herding sheep; being herded to and fro without them knowing where they are going.

Assembling the masses of the army, and throwing them into danger are the responsibility of the general.

Adaptations to the nine grounds, the advantages in defensive and offensive maneuvers, and the patterns of human emotions must be examined.

Generally, the Way of invading is: When troops are deep in enemy ground, they are united; when troops are not deep in enemy ground, they are scattered.

Where you leave your country, and lead the troops across the border into enemy ground, this is called isolated ground. Where there are four sides open, this is called intersecting ground. Where you penetrated deep in enemy ground, this is called critical ground.

Where you penetrated little in enemy ground, this is called marginal ground. Where the back is impassable and the front is narrow, this is called surrounded ground. Where there is nowhere to go, this is called deadly ground.

Therefore,

On isolated ground, I have my troops united.
On marginal ground, I consolidate my troops.
On contentious ground, I hurry my back.
On open ground, I pay attention to our defenses.
On intersecting ground, I strengthen our alliances.
On critical ground, I maintain continuous supply of provisions.
On difficult ground, I press on quickly.
On surrounded ground, I block off openings.
On deadly ground, I show the troops our resolve to fight to the death.

DR. CHAN says:

You are the leader of your health. Strive to be calm and disciplined. You must know how to make changes and be knowledgeable of the nine situations or stages, as well as their strategies and advantages.

1. *Dispersive ground: You must find your ground and focus on what you want for your health.*
2. *Easy ground: When you are here, continue and don't stop.*
3. *Contested ground: Maintain unity & focus, even though you may be tempted to do other unhealthy things.*
4. *Open ground: Know where you are, to get where you want to go.*
5. *Shared ground: Find the right healthcare partners (doctor, nutritionist, etc) to share your healthcare. Family and friends influence your health, share your goals and knowledge.*
6. *Dangerous ground: Beware of running out of resources - financial resources, or physical and mental energy.*

119

7. *Difficult ground*: When in this stage, re-kindle interest in your health, (what is your vision? What are the incentives of being healthy?).

8. *Limited ground*: Use surprise and motivation strategies.

9. *Deadly ground*: Fight and give it your all.

To commit to change, you must understand the different levels of health behavior change and how to deal with them.

Stages of Health Behavior Change

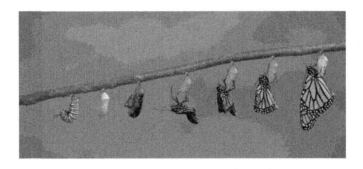

Studies show that people move through a series of stages when making changes. There are certain tasks and principles required at each stage in order to progress to the next stage.

Some of the traits needed to be successful at change are self-efficacy, or the self-confidence needed to make the change, determination or perseverance, and decision-making skills – weighing the pros and cons.

Change takes time. The time needed at each stage is as individual as each person. (Though there is a general amount of time that is usual for the stages.) The stages can be achieved in sequence or the beginning stages can be recycled, due to relapses, until the final stage, termination, is reached.

Pre-contemplation (not ready)

A person is pre-contemplative when they are uninformed and not ready to take action to make a change in the near future (around six months).

Contemplation (getting ready)

People in the contemplation stage are aware of the need to change and are getting ready to take action towards a change in the near future (six months). They are weighing the pros and cons of change. Sometimes people can stay in this stage for an extended period of time, especially if the benefits and costs of taking action are about equal. It can then be characterized as procrastination.

Preparation (ready)

The preparation stage is where people are ready to take action in the immediate future (in one month). They have usually taken some steps toward the action (researched gyms or doctors) and are ready to take the action (join the gym, make the appointment).

Action

People in the action stage have taken specific steps to change their lifestyle (lasting at least six months). Actions for health change include: following a program to stop smoking, lose weight, exercise, following through with an appointment to see a health care provider, following through on preventive testing, etc.

Maintenance

The maintenance stage is when people have followed through and made changes to their lifestyle for over six months. The temptation to relapse is low, but still exists. Studies show maintenance can last anywhere from 6 months to 5 years.

Termination

The termination stage is when the change is complete and has been made for life. There is no need for the old behavior and no temptation for relapse.

Wellness Warrior Actions: Week 10

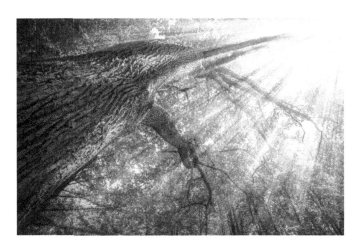

Vision Meditation
- Have your journal ready to record your thoughts after you meditate.
- Sit in a private, quiet, and comfortable place.
- Close your eyes and relax.
- Take a deep breath in and exhale three times to empty the air in your chest (this will start your deep breathing).
- Take a breath for each number and count backwards from 10 to 1, as you relax your body and center yourself. Notice where there is tension and let it go with your breath.
- Think about how your week went. How did you do on the past week's goal or goals?
- Is there anything you would have done differently?
- **For week 10**– Meditate on where you are in relation to your health – on what grounds? What change do you need to make? At what behavioral stage are you in with regard to the change? Are you ready? Getting ready? Taking action?

- Refer back to your healthy vision. Begin to see what it would look like in the future if you followed the stages of change and made positive changes in your health. What would that look like a few months from now, a year from now, 10 years from now? See yourself as very healthy due to the changes you made. What does that look like? What does that feel like?

Journaling
- Write "Week 10" in your journal and record what you accomplished this week in keeping your goal or goals. Write any observations you may have and what you may want to do differently in the future.

This week's goals
- Go through the Nine situations or stages below and write down your thoughts about each stage and how you can use the strategy for your health.

Some examples:
- What do you want for your health?
- What is easy ground for you?
- What are your temptations and how do you plan to maintain focus?
- Who do you want to be and where do you want to go with your health?
- Do you need to find the right healthcare partner (doctor, nutritionist, etc.) Do you need to bring your family and friends on board?
- How are your resources? How can you plan for better financial resources, for physical and mental resources?
- How is your self-talk? How can you keep track and motivate yourself to use positive self-talk?
- Are you battling disease? What else can you do to give it your all?

Nine Situations or Stages

1. _Dispersive ground_: Find your ground - focus on what you want for your health.
2. _Easy ground_: Continue and don't stop.
3. _Contested ground_: Maintain unity & focus, even though you may be tempted to do other unhealthy things.
4. _Open ground_: Unobstructed ground. Know where you are, to get where you want to go.
5. _Shared ground_: Find the right healthcare partners (doctor, nutritionist, etc).
6. _Dangerous ground_: Beware of running out of resources (financial resources, physical and mental energy).
7. _Difficult ground_: When in this stage, re-kindle your interest in your health, (what are the incentives of being healthy?)
8. _Limited ground_: Transitional/vulnerable stage, self-doubt (negative self-talk) – use surprise and motivation.
9. _Deadly ground_: Do or die - fight and give it your all.

What is something that you are thinking of changing? What can you do to move to the next stage of change? Write that out as a goal. Be sure it is a SMART goal. (For example:

- I will research gyms each night after dinner and decide by Friday where I want to join.
- I will call a walking buddy this week and arrange a day and time each week to walk.
- I will pack a salad for lunch every night after dinner, starting next Monday.
- I will meditate every day for 10 minutes when I come home from work.

Try to attach your goals to an anchor – something you already do consistently (wake up, eat breakfast, take a shower, go to work, eat lunch, come home from work, eat dinner, go to bed). (e.g., After I take a shower each day, I will do 10 minutes of stretching and toning exercises. After lunch on Sundays, I will make my list of healthy menus for the week and then go grocery shopping.) Make sure your goals are SMART goals.

S – Specific: What exactly do you want to do? Clearly define your goal.

M – Measurable: How can you measure and track progress?

A – Attainable: Can you achieve it in the time frame?

R – Relevant: Is it relevant to your long-term goals?

T – Time bound: When will you take action? Time sensitive goals are more likely to be achieved than a loose thought of action without an end time attached to it.

"In health, become skilled at preventing disease. You don't want to fight disease, you want to disorganize disease."

~ Dr. Kevin Chan

WEEK 11

HEALTH ENVIRONMENTAL

ATTACKS

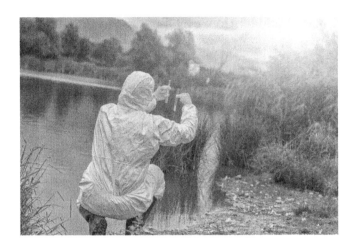

According to Sun Tzu we should use the environment to our advantage to avoid attacks.

He terms this chapter "Fire Attacks," but the broader meaning is: environmental attacks.

Healthcare providers are warriors on the front line of environmental medicine. Environmental medicine and environmental heath are concerned with natural and man-made environmental disease factors, such as: air pollution, noise pollution, chemicals used in farming, chemicals and metals used in products, chemicals and metals in the natural environment (radon – a naturally occurring radioactive gas, lead – a toxic heavy metal, etc.), asthma triggers, radiation and electro-magnetic fields, carbon dioxide, and more. These disease factors are considered a toxic burden on the body.

There are many toxic affronts to humans in today's world. Thousands of chemicals can end up in the body, due to pesticides, chemicals in processed food and household products, and in the environment around us. Noise and excess artificial light can also create an adverse environment for health.

Large toxic exposures do not occur that frequently. It is everyday exposure, chronic toxin exposure, that accumulates and creates a total body toxic burden. This burden, in turn, disrupts systems in the body and can cause disease. The main systems that are disrupted are the: hormonal, nervous, and detoxification systems. But these disruptions then affect other systems in the body as well.

The external environment is having a serious impact on people's immune system. Due to the chronic toxic burden, doctors are seeing more patients with what is now termed – Irritable Immune Syndrome. Their immune systems react to the foreign substances in a confused way - in a hypo-state of underperforming or becoming desensitized; or a hyper-state, whereby the immune system becomes overly activated and sensitive to toxins. Due to this phenomenon, autoimmune disorders are on the rise. They have tripled in the last few decades.

Climate change is an important factor in current medicine. Because of the rise in temperatures, doctors are seeing more patients with allergies, which trigger autoimmune responses.

Some conditions, which studies show are strongly linked to environmental conditions, are:
- Asthma
- Autism
- Autoimmune diseases (e.g. Lupus)
- Cancers
- Lung Diseases
- Obesity
- Parkinson's Disease
- Hormonal and Reproductive Health

Quality preventive care addresses these diseases, and how to treat them, by incorporating environmental and integrative medicine best practices.

SUN TZU said:

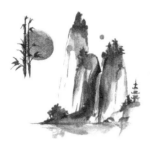

There are five kinds of fire attacks: One, burning personnel; two, burning provisions; three, burning equipment; four, burning stores; five, burning weapons.

Using fire attacks depends on proper conditions. Equipment for fire attacks must be available beforehand.

There are appropriate seasons for using fire attacks, and appropriate days for raising fires. The appropriate season is when the weather is dry; the appropriate day is when the moon is at Chi, Pi, I, or Chen. These four days are when there are rising winds.

Generally, in fire attacks, you must respond according to the five changes of fire: If the fires are set inside enemy camp, you must respond quickly outside the enemy camp; if the fires are set but the enemy is calm, then wait, do not attack. Let the fire reach its height, and follow up if you can, stay if you cannot.

If the fire attack can be set outside, without relying on the inside, set it when the time is right. If the fire is set upwind, do not attack downwind. If it is windy all during the day, the wind will stop at night. The army must know the five changes of fire, to be able to calculate the appropriate days.

DR. CHAN says:

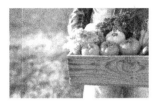

Sun Tzu calls this chapter fire attacks, but the broader meaning is the environment or environmental attacks and what we can do about them. I have listed the nine common environments that affect our health.

The Nine Environments:
1. *You – Your core that is unchanging.*
2. *Body – Physical health, energy.*
3. *Self – Personality, gifts, talents, strengths, emotions.*
4. *Spiritual – Connection to higher source, love and self.*
5. *Nature – Natural beauty, seasons, the cycle of life.*
6. *Physical – Home and office environment, furnishings, equipment, technology.*
7. *Financial – Money, investments, budgeting, insurance.*
8. *Network – Community, strategic partners, customers.*
9. *Relationships – Family, friends, colleagues, support network.*

Present day environmental attacks are many. If you want to achieve optimal wellness you must strive to eliminate and reduce your exposure to environmental toxins.

Good nutrition is important and can help detoxify the liver, kidneys, and skin. Eating a wide range of vegetables is essential in delivering micro nutrients and vitamins. Eat organic whenever possible. Eliminate processed foods and wheat flour, and limit dairy and alcohol. Wild caught fatty fish such as salmon is recommended, as well as meat that is antibiotic and synthetic hormone free.

Make sure your water intake is optimal and you exercise for good circulation and to filter and remove toxins.

Environmental toxins can lead to imbalanced hormones. I suggest you have your hormones checked. Imbalanced hormones can lead to several conditions, including: chronic fatigue, thyroid issues, metabolic syndrome (a precursor to diabetes), and more.

Read labels to be sure the products you are using in your home, such as cleaning products, as well as personal hygiene products, do not contain harmful chemicals.

Be aware of the noise and lights in your environments. Change any fluorescent lighting you may have. We are children of the sun. The sun is full spectrum lighting and our body chemistry depends on it. Fluorescent lighting is very limited spectrum lighting and has been known to cause several health related issues, including: migraine headaches, eye strain, anxiety, depression, sleep problems, endocrine disruption, immune problems, obesity, and more.

Go outside for at least 15-20 minutes a day to get some natural vitamin D.

Test for radon in your home and office.
Be aware of the toxins around you to protect your health.

SUN TZU said:

Those who use fire to assist in attacks are intelligent, those who use water to assist in attacks are powerful. Water can be used to cut off the enemy, but cannot be used to plunder.

If one gains victory in battle and is successful in attacks, but does not exploit those achievements, it is disastrous. This is called waste and delay.

Therefore, I say the wise general thinks about it, and the good general executes it.

If it is not advantageous, do not move; if there is no gain, do not use troops; if there is no danger, do not do battle.

The ruler may not move his army out of anger; the general may not do battle out of wrath.

If it is advantageous, move; if it is not advantageous, stop.

Those angry will be happy again, and those wrathful will be cheerful again, but a destroyed nation cannot exist again, the dead cannot be brought back to life.

Therefore, the enlightened ruler is prudent, the good general is cautious. This is the Way of securing the nation, and preserving the army.

DR. CHAN says:

Those who use the environment to their advantage are intelligent.

The wise person thinks about their nine environments, and makes a move when advantageous. Timing is important.

Those who are enlightened know the Way. This is also in accordance with the principles of Feng Shui, an ancient system of harmonizing with the environment, and QMDJ (Qi Men Dun Jia), an ancient Chinese tactical system that teaches timing is everything.

Feng Shui and QMDJ

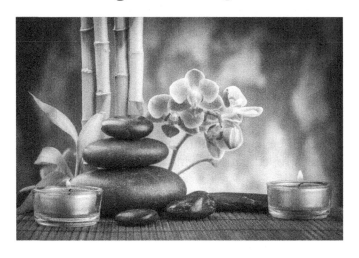

Feng Shui is the ancient system of harmonizing with one's environment. It is one of the five arts of Chinese Metaphysics. Through calculations and formulas, Feng Shui works with the life force energy that binds the universe, earth, and humanity together. This energy is called "qi" and is the basis of Chinese Metaphysics.

The main principle of Feng Shui is to align the environment with yin and yang forces so that there is a flow of qi. The goal is to have an environment that promotes calmness, happiness, and mindfulness.

Ancient Feng Shui practices used astronomy for calculations. They used the heavens to ascertain earthly positions. The magnetic compass was invented for Feng Shui and follows the same ancient Chinese calculations developed centuries ago.

Some of the modern day principles of Feng Shui are:

Positive energy - *Creating positive energy is the main reason for Feng Shui. Above all, positive energy needs to be maintained when creating and aligning an environment. This includes a healthy environment.*

A sense of balance - *The yin and yang of Feng Shui can be seen in the balance of objects. This can present in many forms in the special aspects of objects - textures, symmetry, and colors play an important role in balancing an environment.*

An appreciation for beauty – *Creating beautiful places can include symmetry (of rooms, furniture, outside spaces, etc.), objects, or something as simple as a small bunch of flowers placed strategically so you can view it from several places. Celebrating beauty invites positive energy.*

An expression of love – *Your environment should reflect a love of self and those people and things you love, as well as a love of your environment. This mindfulness of your environment will promote mindfulness in your life.*

Supportive of your dreams – *Feng Shui includes you, the universe, and your future self. Your environment should support and reflect the big dreams that are already unfolding. Feng Shui creates a space where you are living "as if" the dreams are coming to fruition. It ensures that there is alignment between the things you want and the things that are manifested in the objects you see every day.*

Qi Men Dun Jia (QMDJ)

Sun Tzu teaches to do the right thing, QMDJ shows how to do it the right way at the right time.

The ancient art of strategizing and forecasting your future, QMDJ consists of various aspects of Chinese metaphysics. It is a way to be mindful, by staying in the present and analyzing the decisions for your future.

QMDJ is a tool that gives you a way to analyze and map out the best options for you. It uses the doctrines of yin and yang, the five elements, eight trigrams, and others. It is the oldest form of Feng Shui. In current terms, QMDJ is Feng Shui for your life in that it promotes mindfulness. Creating the future you want depends on being mindful of the decisions that are best for you.

QMDJ uses a chart to map out the best options for you at a given time. In ancient times they used a complicated system to navigate time, space (environment), matter and event, as well as the year, month, day and hour. Today the charts are computerized and tell you on any given day what are the best options for you. The key to QMDJ is always timing. QMDJ is developed on the concept that actions are most beneficial when it is the right time to do them.

You may be in circumstances beyond your control, but QMDJ will aid you in dealing with problems in your life and help you take control of future outcomes.

Indeed, QMDJ can be considered as the tactical complement to Sun Tzu's the Art of War.

Wellness Warrior Actions – Week 11

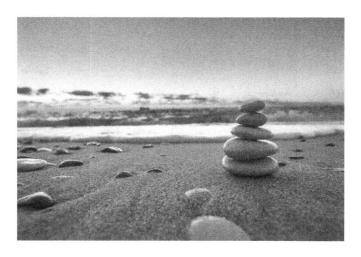

Vision Meditation

- Have your journal ready to record your thoughts after you meditate.
- Sit in a private, quiet, and comfortable place.
- Close your eyes and relax.
- Take a deep breath in and exhale three times to empty the air in your chest (this will start your deep breathing).
- Take a breath for each number and count backwards from 10 to 1, as you relax your body and center yourself. Notice where there is tension and let it go with your breath.
- Think about how your week went. How did you do on the past week's goal or goals?
- Is there anything you would have done differently?
- **For week 11**– Meditate on your environment. Visualize your environments and see where you have toxins or a toxic environment. Visualize your home and work environments. What feelings do they promote?
- Refer back to your healthy vision. Begin to see what it would look like in the future if you made changes in your environment to eliminate toxins and create a positive, healthy environment. What would that look like a few

months from now, a year from now, 10 years from now? See yourself as very healthy due to your actions. What does that look like? What does that feel like?

Journaling

- Write "Week 11" in your journal and record what you accomplished this week in keeping your goal or goals. Write any observations you may have and what you may want to do differently in the future.

This week's goals

- Write down the environmental toxins that you believe you can eliminate or reduce and how you would do that. Is it your diet (e.g., eliminating processed foods and buying organic when possible), your water (e.g., purchasing a filtering system or filtering pitcher), cleaning products or personal hygiene products you use (e.g., purchase natural products)? Do you have fluorescent lighting in your home or work? Pick one area that you will start to change this week and write it as a goal (e.g., This week I will eliminate processed foods from my diet. I will plan weekly menus that don't include processed food. I will not buy any processed foods and will substitute with fresh whole foods. I will also go through the pantry and throw out any processed foods. Or – this week I will bring in a lamp for my desk at work, and not turn on the overhead fluorescent light.
- Go over the principals of Feng Shui (below) and write down your feelings about your home and work environments. How could you improve them to reflect the principles of Feng Shui (listed below)? Write down one thing you could do this week to promote "qi" in your home or office. Write it as a goal (e.g., this week I will print the family photo I love, frame it, and take it to work for my desk. Or – this weekend I will work in the garden or clean the patio or declutter a

room, and then relax and appreciate the beauty of the space. Or – this week I will paint a room a color I love, that makes me feel calm or gives me a feeling of positive energy.

Be sure to write your goals as SMART goals.

S – Specific: What exactly do you want to do? Clearly define your goal.

M – Measurable: How can you measure and track progress?

A – Attainable: Can you achieve it in the time frame?

R – Relevant: Is it relevant to your long-term goals?

T – Time bound: When will you take action? Time sensitive goals are more likely to be achieved than a loose thought of action without an end time attached to it.

Modern Day Principals of Feng Shui

Positive energy - Creating positive energy is the main reason for Feng Shui. Above all, positive energy needs to be maintained when creating and aligning an environment. This includes a healthy environment.

A sense of balance - The yin and yang of Feng Shui can be seen in the balance of objects. This can present in many forms in the special aspects of objects - textures, symmetry, and colors play an important role in balancing an environment.

An appreciation for beauty – Creating beautiful places can include symmetry (of rooms, furniture, outside spaces, etc.), objects, or something as simple as a small bunch of flowers placed strategically so you can view it from several places. Celebrating beauty invites positive energy.

An expression of love – Your environment should reflect a love of self and those people and things you love, as well as a love of your environment. This mindfulness of your environment will promote mindfulness in your life.

Supportive of your dreams – Feng Shui includes you, the universe and your future self. Your environment should support and reflect the big dreams that are already unfolding. Feng Shui creates a space where you are living "as if" the dreams are coming to fruition. It ensures that there is alignment between the things you want and the things that are manifested in the objects you see every day.

"If it is advantageous, move; if it is not advantageous, stop. Those angry will be happy again, and those wrathful will be cheerful again, but a destroyed nation cannot exist again, the dead cannot be brought back to life. Therefore, the enlightened ruler is prudent, the good general is cautious. "

~ Sun Tzu

WEEK 12

HEALTH INFORMATION SOURCES

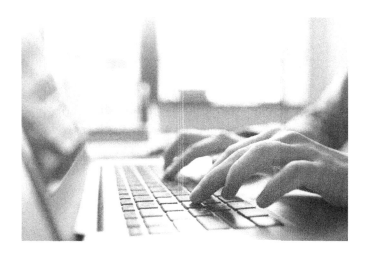

Sun Tzu teaches that information is key for successful strategy. All other strategies and skills rest on the foundation of good information. Sun Tzu terms this chapter "spies," but the broader interpretation is - knowledge or information. He breaks knowledge into five sources that correlate with the Five Elements of Strategic Analysis:

1. Timely/trending sources (Heaven)
2. Local/body (Ground)
3. Competitive sources (Method/Law)
4. Inside, personality traits you have (Leader)
5. Messenger/ information sources that bring about your mindset or reality (Philosophy/Way)

In regard to your health, you need to gather information so you can take care of yourself, but how do you know it's the right information? Use Sun Tzu's principles to collect information to be sure you are collecting quality information.

SUN TZU said:

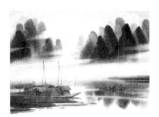

Generally, raising an army of a hundred thousand and advancing it a thousand kilometers, the expenses to the people and the nation's resources are one thousand gold pieces a day.

Those in commotion internally and externally, those exhausted on the roads, and those unable to do their daily work are seven hundred thousand families.

Two sides remain in standoff for several years in order to do battle for a decisive victory on a single day.

Yet one refusing to outlay a hundred pieces of gold and thereby does not know the enemy's situation is the height of inhumanity. This one is not the general of the people, a help to the ruler, or the master of victory.

What enables the enlightened rulers and good generals to conquer the enemy at every move and achieve extraordinary success is foreknowledge.

Foreknowledge cannot be elicited from ghosts and spirits; it cannot be inferred from comparison of previous events, or from the calculations of the heavens, but must be obtained from people who have knowledge of the enemy's situation.

Therefore there are five kinds of spies used: Local spies, internal spies, double spies, dead spies, and living spies.

When all five are used, and no one knows their Way, it is called the divine organization, and is the ruler's treasure.

For local spies, we use the enemy's people. For internal spies we use the enemy's officials. For double spies we use the enemy's spies. For dead spies we use agents to spread misinformation to the enemy. For living spies, we use agents to return with reports.

DR. CHAN says:

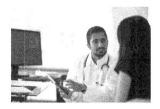

Information and knowledge is key to your health strategy, especially foreknowledge or preventive information.

You need to collect information so you can take care of yourself. How can you gather information? How can you be sure it's trustworthy? According to Sun Tzu you need to gather the right information the right way, and there are five ways to gather the right information:

Timely/trending sources (Heaven) *– Gather up-to-date information from health organizations, news, journals, newsletters, and your healthcare providers.*

Local/body (Ground) *– Gather information from knowledgeable healthcare providers. Gather from friends, family, and people you know who have good information or can tell you where to go to get quality information (e.g., refer a good health care provider, etc.)*

Competitive sources (Method) – *You are competing against disease, therefore, you need to consistently gather information about your health and the healthiest lifestyle you can live.*

Inside, your personality traits (Leader) – *Gather information to keep yourself not only physically healthy and strong, but also emotionally and mentally strong, so you can be a leader for your health and your life.*

Messenger/ information sources that bring about your mindset or reality (Philosophy) – *Watch out for media sources, they are not always accurate. You have to do your own research. Follow sources you know to be credible.*

SUN TZU said:

Therefore, of those close to the army, none is closer than spies, no reward more generously given, and no matter in greater secrecy.

Only the wisest ruler can use spies; only the most benevolent and upright general can use spies, and only the most alert and observant person can get the truth using spies. It is subtle, subtle!

There is nowhere that spies cannot be used.

If a spy's activities are leaked before they are to begin, the spy and those who know should be put to death.

Generally, if you want to attack an army, besiege a walled city, assassinate individuals, you must know the identities of the defending generals, assistants, associates, gate guards, and officers.

You must have spies seek and learn them. You must seek enemy spies. Bribe them, and instruct and retain them. Therefore, double spies can be obtained and used.

From their knowledge, you can obtain local and internal spies. From their knowledge, the dead spies can spread misinformation to the enemy. From their knowledge, our living spies can be used as planned. The ruler must know these five kinds of espionage.

This knowledge depends on the double spies. Therefore, you must treat them with the utmost generosity.

In ancient times, the rise of the Yin dynasty was due to I Chih, who served the house of Hsia; the rise of the Chou dynasty was due to Lu Ya, who served the house of Yin.

Therefore, enlightened rulers and good generals who are able to obtain intelligent agents as spies are certain for great achievements.

This is essential for warfare, and what the army depends on to move.

DR. CHAN says:

Optimal health depends on good information. Those who have access to quality health information are better armed against disease. You must have the right information to make informed decisions. Gather your information and use it wisely, to eliminate any costly mistakes.

Wellness Warrior Actions – Week 12

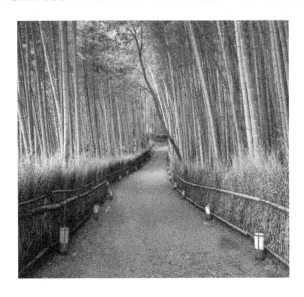

Vision Meditation

- Have your journal ready to record your thoughts after your meditate.
- Sit in a private, quiet, and comfortable place.
- Close your eyes and relax.
- Take a deep breath in and exhale three times to empty the air in your chest (this will start your deep breathing).
- Take a breath for each number and count backwards from 10 to 1, as you relax your body and center yourself. Notice where there is tension and let it go with your breath.
- Think about how your week went. How did you do on the past week's goal or goals?
- Is there anything you would have done differently?
- **For week 12** – Meditate on how you get your quality health information. Are your sources the best you can get? What information do you need? Where will you get it?
- Refer back to your healthy vision. Begin to see what it would look like in the future if you consistently had good sources of health information. What would that look like a

few months from now, a year from now, 10 years from now? See yourself as very healthy due to the health information sources you have. What does that look like? What does that feel like?

Journaling

- Write "Week 11" in your journal and record what you accomplished this week in keeping your goal or goals. Write any observations you may have and what you may want to do differently in the future.

This Week's Goals

- Set a goal of gathering quality health information you can use. Follow the five strategies and come up with a list of resources you can use.

Five Information Strategies

1. Timely/trending sources (Heaven) –Gather up-to-date information from health organizations, news, journals, newsletters, and your healthcare providers.
2. Local/body (Ground) – Gather information from healthcare providers for quality information. Gather from friends, family, and people you know who have good information or can tell you where to go to get quality information (refer good health care providers, etc.)
3. Competitive sources (Method) – You are competing against disease, therefore, you need to consistently gather information about your health and living the healthiest lifestyle you can.
4. Inside, your personality traits (Leader) – Gather information to keep yourself not only physically healthy and strong, but also emotionally and mentally strong, so you can be a leader for your health and your life.
5. Messenger/ information sources that bring about your mindset or reality (Philosophy) – Watch out for media

sources, they are not always accurate. You have to do your own research. Follow sources you know to be credible.

"Being healthy is a way of living."

~ Dr. Kevin Chan

CONCLUSION

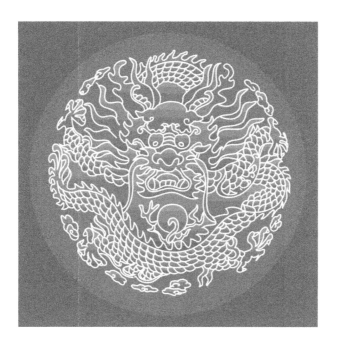

As people live longer, more of the population has one or more chronic diseases.

The current medical system works well for acute care, but is not a good model for chronic disease. Many scientists and medical professionals believe the current model needs to be changed because it is inadequate in dealing with the mushrooming population that has complex chronic diseases like autoimmune disease, diabetes, arthritis, kidney disease, and cancers.

To change the system, we must first change the way we think about health and medicine. As you now know, Sun Tzu's writings and philosophy is a system of how to think about anything strategically. Many people have used it as the basis for successful economic, business, and professional sports models. But now you can see that

Sun Tzu's philosophy can be used as an effective medical and health model. His model is designed to study a complex system in a simple way, which is the perfect foundation for a new health care system – Strategic Integrative Medicine.

Strategic Integrative Medicine is a progressive style of medicine that incorporates the best practices of integrative, functional, and mind-body medicine in the framework of Sun Tzu's strategic system with the scientific application of ancient metaphysical principles.

Integrative medicine addresses the full range of physical, emotional, mental, social, spiritual and environmental influences that affect a person's health. It considers the patient's unique conditions, needs, and circumstances, and combines alternative medicine and therapies with conventional medicine to diagnose and treat their disease. It focuses on prevention rather than treating disease and also promotes a strong patient-physician relationship.

Functional Medicine is a form of integrative medicine that uses a systems approach to address the root causes of ill health and disease, many times in its preventive stage. It focuses on the interactions of the body's systems with the environment and with each other. Through biochemical diagnostic testing, to evaluate how systems are functioning, functional medicine discovers and treats the underlying causes of disease and imbalances.

META-Medicine is based on mind-body medicine and is the science of the bio-psycho-social connection. It is based on scientific evidence emerging from more than 30 years of brain scans and research that there is a body-mind-social connection that affects health.

The foundations of Sun Tzu's teachings give us the strategies for Strategic Integrative Medicine. They provide the compass that tells us where we are in our health and the tools to show us how to get where we want to go. In summary, they are:

The Five Elements of Strategic Health Analysis:

1. **Way** (Mindset)
   This is your belief system, your philosophy, your mission, your values.

   How healthy do you want to be? What do you believe? What is your mission?

   Your beliefs will propel you. You need to know your beliefs and values; they will lead you to a healthy life.

2. **Heaven** (Mind)
   Heaven pertains to things you cannot easily control: weather, climate, the seasons, timing, and trends. In health it also relates to aging. You cannot control getting older and you cannot easily control changes in your body. Ask yourself – how do I deal with aging? What is my plan? It also pertains to your emotional wellbeing as opposed to your physical wellbeing. It pertains to integrative medicine as opposed to conventional medicine.

3. **Ground** (Body)
   This is your terrain – your body and state of physical being. It's where you have more immediate control. It's where you fight. What are you fighting for? Your health and longevity. What are you struggling with right now in your health?

4. **Leader** (Character)
   The general or leader makes good decisions. Leadership pertains to things like character, personality, and attitude. Do you have what it takes to be a good leader for your health? What do you need to do or work on to be a good leader? If you are a leader of your health you must be:

- Wise – You must be knowledgeable about your health. Study health and how you can be healthier.
- Trustworthy – Find good health practitioners who are trustworthy. Then do your part to be trustworthy too.
- Benevolent – You must have compassion and care for yourself. Health is very much about self-care.
- Courageous – You must be brave and take the actions needed to be healthy.
- Disciplined – Be accountable for your health. Do your part – study, have a plan, keep to your plan and follow-through.

5. **Law** (Systems)

Systems you have set up to carry out a situation.

What systems do you have in place to keep you on your plan to becoming healthier?

The Four Healthcare Environments

1. **Level Ground,** (Stable, Neutral, Predictable) – Ideal environment for maintaining good health.
2. **Marshes** (Soft, Unpredictable) – Diseases
3. **Water** (Fluid, Unstable) – New trends in healthcare and drugs.
4. **Mountains** (Tilted, Uneven) – Doctors, healthcare system, insurance.

Level ground, is the ideal environment for good health. It is a stable environment to maintain good health and use the advantages of the other environments to position yourself. It includes: integrative medicine, functional medicine, and mind-body medicine. Level ground is easy to navigate so you can position yourself for success, staying healthy and avoiding disease.

Marshes and swamps represent disease. You want to move quickly through swamps, (disease), because you don't want it to develop into something chronic, because it takes a toll on your body, and can be costly in many ways.

Water is not stable. It represents current trends in medicine: current nutrition, exercise, medication, and testing recommendations. These are trends that are always changing.

Mountains are uneven, complicated terrains, with many variations. They are healthcare providers, the current healthcare system, and insurers. They can be hard to navigate and range from small organizations and practices to large bureaucracies.

The Six Dimensions of Health Positioning

The six positions help you know where you are going at any given time. You should know where you are in relation to disease. Are you moving forward, waiting, attacking, or defending?

Areas/Distance:

1. **Spread out – Far:** In this position where many things are spread out or far away, you need to handle tasks without overextending yourself or spreading yourself too thin. If you do overextend yourself, you will be surprised by disease.

2. **Constricted – Close, unity, focused:** The constricted position is one that requires focus and unity. If you cannot stay focused, in this position you will usually have self-doubts, which will lead to self-destruction or self-sabotage.

Obstruction/Obstacles:

3. **Wide-open/Accessible – Easy to get to:** When you are in a wide-open position, things are easily accessible and it's easy to maneuver. But, you can become clumsy and then potentially outmaneuvered by disease. Therefore, you must take care not to be clumsy when things are easy.

4. **Barricaded – Hard to get to:** If you are barricaded, it is a good position because it will be hard for disease to get to you, and easy to defend. Therefore, you must be organized. If you are disorganized, then disease can besiege you.

Dangers/Holding power:
5. Entangling – Difficult to leave: When you are in an entangled position, it is difficult to leave, therefore you must be disciplined and do what needs to be done. If you are not disciplined, you could be hurt.
6. Supportive – Don't want to leave: A supportive position can be a very good position unless you are not knowledgeable and don't know what you are doing. You need to be knowledgeable in order to take a supportive position against disease.

The Nine Stages of Health Situations

1. **Dispersive ground:** This is a state of scattered conditions. You may be scattered or you may have several areas of health concerns, often triggered by unexpected health events, or several healthcare providers. You must find your ground and focus on what you want for your health.

2. **Easy ground:** You can make progress without struggle. When you are here, continue and don't stop.

3. **Contested ground:** This is where you must engage ill health in competition for power. Maintain unity & focus, even though you may be tempted to do other unhealthy things.

4. **Open ground:** You have unobstructed conditions. Know where you are, so you can get where you want to go.

5. **Shared ground:** You share your healthcare and optimal health with healthcare providers, family and friends. Find the right healthcare partners - doctor, nutritionist, etc. - to share

your healthcare. Family and friends influence your health, so share your goals and knowledge.

6. **Dangerous ground:** Conditions are not supporting your health, or you are not supporting your health. Beware of running out of resources - financial resources, or physical and mental energy.

7. **Difficult ground:** Things are not easy. You are having struggles in your life and/or health. When in this stage, re-kindle interest in your health. What is your vision? What are the incentives of being healthy?

8. **Limited ground:** This can be a transitional or vulnerable stage that may include self-doubt and negative self-talk. Use motivational and inspirational strategies that surprise and work for you.

9. **Deadly ground:** You are in the clutches of disease and it is do or die. Fight and give it your all.

Strategic Health Innovation

Sun Tzu translates innovation to mean something akin to momentum - the blending of standard strategies and new strategies in order to win. We interpret this as innovation. Innovation in health care is the standard strategy - conventional medicine - combined with the new strategy - Strategic Integrative Medicine.

Anything you do in life requires innovation if you want to be successful; so it is in healthcare. Start with conventional medicine to engage, but use integrative medicine to innovate, to gain momentum, and achieve victory – optimal health.

Complementary Opposites in Healthcare – Yin and Yang

Yin and Yang is the bedrock of Chinese philosophy. They represent complementary opposites that are the perfect balance of nature. They are opposite, yet interconnected through forces that complement each other. We must not forget their mutual interdependence; you cannot have one without the other. Day and night, dark and light.

Health Information through knowledge

Sun Tzu teaches that through the complementary opposites of weakness and strength we are able to turn challenges into opportunities. The yin and yang of healthcare is: if extreme in one area, it gives rise to the opposite. (Yin is only yin when compared to yang. Yang is only yang when compared to yin.) Competition only exists in the context of comparison, comparing your old self with your current and future self.

Sun Tzu compares knowledge and ignorance with strength and weakness. He encourages focusing strengths on the weakness of the opposition, so you can exploit the opposition. In relation to your healthcare – stay focused and know your strengths and weaknesses. Use your strengths by bringing in experts to attack any weaknesses in your health.

My Hope

These strategies are the basis for Strategic Integrative Medicine, and have served me and my patients well. It is my sincere hope that this book will INSPIRE you to take ACTION to strategize your health decisions, redirect your health destiny, and serve as the beginning of a new philosophy in health and medicine.

ACKNOWLEDGMENTS

I would like to acknowledge Sonshi.com for the Sun Tzu translation used in this book, and for the work they do to educate people about Sun Tzu. A special acknowledgement to Gary Gagliardi for his friendship and his works on Sun Tzu, especially *The Amazing Secrets of Sun Tzu's The Art of War,* which helped to form the framework of this book.

Thank you to Penny Breen Aleo for her writing and editing contributions to *The Art of Health.* And last, but certainly not least, thank you to Nurse Practitioner Virginia Greene, a dedicated member of my practice, who consistently encouraged me to write my book.

ABOUT THE AUTHORS

Dr. Kevin Chan is one of the nation's foremost physicians in the integration of Eastern and Western medicine, and a sought-after speaker. He is the founder of Strategic Integrative Medicine, also known as Health Destiny Management, which is a preventive style of medicine that incorporates the best practices of integrative, functional, and mind-body medicine, with Chinese strategic and metaphysical principles.

Dr. Chan is a board-certified physician, as well as a specialist in lipidology, age management, integrative, and classical Chinese medicine. He is also a licensed trainer for the Science of Strategy Institute. Dr. Chan has a private practice in Phoenix, Arizona.

Penny Breen Aleo is a health, wellness, and medical writer and co-author. Her writing focuses on progressive health issues that encourage people toward greater health and wellbeing. Ms. Aleo has been a health writer for over 25 years and also holds certifications in personal training, nutrition, and health and wellness coaching.

Made in the USA
Las Vegas, NV
09 December 2022

61593022R00098